Will "Power" Byron
Superfood Awakening

AuthorHouse™
1663 Liberty Drive, Suite 200
Bloomington, IN 47403
www.authorhouse.com
Phone: 1-800-839-8640

© 2010 Will Power. All rights reserved.

No part of this book may be reproduced, stored in a retrieval system, or transmitted by any means without the written permission of the author.

First published by AuthorHouse 1/28/2010

ISBN: 978-1-4389-4274-2 (sc)

Printed in the United States of America
Bloomington, Indiana

This book is printed on acid-free paper.

DISCLAIMER: Information within this book is for educational purposes only. Statements about the efficacy of products mentioned have not been evaluated by the U.S. Food & Drug Administration. The products discussed have been used by the author and all results experienced are true, however, suggestions are not intended to diagnose, treat, cure, or prevent any disease.

Chapter One – The Roots

The superfood train arrived in my life several years ago while attending a T.Harv Ecker event and I believe it has taken me to a new level of consciousness as to how I think and feel about what I eat. David Wolfe was a speaker at the event and he made such a great impression on me. He clarified many years of blurred understanding of nutritional concepts that I had learned.

There are currently many forces that control our actions as to what we currently eat and how we eat it, but as we begin to understand the power of superfoods and slowly add them to our diet, we have the ability to be driven by natural life force energies, as we were from the early beginnings of civilization. Over time, mankind has been driven by many powerful forces. There is perhaps nothing more powerful than an individual's belief in a higher power or spirit. We are taught to believe in the existence of a higher being at a young age, and at times, the miracles and tragedies that we witness daily make it seem inevitable that this Supreme Being exists. How else can we explain coincidence, luck, and unexplained phenomena? How do we digest the teachings and beliefs of our ancestors? For me, the closest thing to an explanation comes when I look at the sun. I can see it, feel it, and I see the consequences of its actions every time I see a living plant or animal.

There are so many different schools of thought when it comes to who we are, when it all started, and when it will all end. Our existence, in fact, is defined in many ways across different cultures. One thing that has become clear to me over the past few years is that there is one undeniable fact that is universal to just about all of us. That fact extends beyond all borders, religions, cultures, and civilizations, and that fact is that we are what we eat and that what we eat is primarily created by the sun. I am reminded of this fact every time I look up at the sun. That glowing light in the sky called our sun is responsible for ongoing life on earth, as it provides the warmth and energy for our plants to grow and feed us. It has done this for billions of years. The sun implants life force energy in our foods, which is then transferred to us when we eat the fruits and vegetables which have captured its light—just as the first living organisms, phytoplankton, did billions of years ago.

In fact, I believe I witness a glimpse of this life force energy every time I look at a Kirlian photograph of living foods. When I first saw these Kirlian images of raw food side by side with cooked food, I felt that some of the mysteries of those higher powers had been cleared up. If there was ever an attempt for those higher powers to impress upon me their existence, it was that very day as I was looking at those images. A Kirlian photograph captures the strength of the living energy field around a photographed object. You can see the light around the edges of a plant leaf or around a living hand or finger. For me, that proof of how important the sun is to creating life force energy in our foods and how important it is that every living cell in our body relies on nourishing itself with that energy was the beginning of my superfood awakening.

Regardless of how it all began, in the end, it doesn't really matter as long as you spiritually grow the way that is best for yourself and mankind. The undeniable fact is that the sun and the earth are made up of mostly the same elements as we are, such as hydrogen, oxygen, carbon, sodium, iron, sulfur, magnesium, etc., and one would not exist without the other. I was never one to dwell on or fight about who was the creator of our solar system five billion years ago. I only have control of my own life in the present. What I know of the past is what is written and what I can see with my own eyes. I don't know how much of what is written is true or not true, but I can see with my eyes and feel with my skin the strength of the sun and how it keeps me alive. So for me, the sun is at least one higher power which I believe is responsible for our current and future existence, at a minimum. The bigger universe outside of our galaxy has even more suns and is till this day being studied and written about. We are always trying to make sense of it. Coming to the realization that we have the power to control our thoughts and well-being by accepting the power of the sun, we can move to a place of a true superfood awakening. We do this by accepting the power that the sun puts in every living organism, including ourselves.

A superfood awakening is an awakening which comes about by our accepting the notion that we are what we eat, drink, and think, and that by eating organic, raw, nutrient-dense, plant based foods and thinking stress-free organic thoughts, we are giving our cells the life force energy that our cells need to flourish and smile. It is that moment when you take control of your lifestyle and stop putting band-aids on your problems in the form of diets, blaming others, relying on what doctors are telling you, and giving your body permission to heal itself.

This superfood awakening will not come easily to everyone because many people suffer from addictions which effect their actions, are exposed to advertising thousands of times a day, are taught and forced to believe what their ancestors believed, traditionally and habitually eat certain foods, and trust those who are supposed to be helping us make better decisions.

Many of us have a story to tell of how we came to be. There are skeletons in the closet, and unfortunate circumstances in our families and our health; and certainly, many of us have what we feel are perfect lives. I want to share my story because I believe many parts of it will have at least one similarity to your own. I want to help everyone achieve their own superfood awakening, because once you do, I believe you will be on your way to living a longer, more enjoyable life. Having a superfood awakening changes your lifestyle and therefore your habits, which control your everyday actions. It is what is needed for you to experience true change. A diet is a one-time prescription. It is like putting a Band-Aid on a leaky hose instead of buying a new hose. I want my book to inspire at least one person—hopefully, more. I realize that not everyone will be able to single-handedly be able to change the world, but what if you could change the life of just one person, or two? There are people out there who are looking for answers. I am going to lead you down a path that was more of a journey for me. This path is one that leads to great health; and as far as I'm concerned, if the journey you choose for your own life does not lead you to great health, you may have chosen the wrong path.

What is the reason I wrote this book?

I have written this book because I have been told my whole life that I should write a book and I feel that now is the time to share the gift I have been giving. As experiences came and went for me, the people who told me I needed to share my gift grew. I then realized upon having my own awakening that many who needed to hear the story would never hear it. The forces of false messages out there are much greater than many of us can imagine. There are doctors with good and bad intentions who are trying to make a living doing what they were taught to do in medical school, there are corporations trying to satisfy their shareholders, and there are parents and grandparents teaching us what they were taught. It reminds me of the story of the woman who always cut the end of the ham off before she put it in the roasting pan. Her daughter asked why she always cut the ends off. The mom said, "Well, my mother always cut the ends off." So they both went to the grandparents' house and wanted to know why she always cut the ends off, and the grandmother replied, "So it would fit in the pan."

I have also written this book because I have accomplished things in my life that others want to accomplish. For instance, here are some of the benefits I have gained from eating primarily raw, organic, living, plant-based superfoods. I have lowered my cholesterol by seventy-five points. I have gotten rid of various stages of arthritis which annoyed me for eight years. I have lost forty pounds. I have lowered my resting heart rate from 59 to 36. I have lowered my blood pressure from 140/90 to 110/60. I have begun to start enjoying life again to its fullest by being able to compete for the first time in years. I have brought key test results into alignment, such as thyroid, neurotransmitters, key minerals, and nutrient levels. I have lowered heavy metal toxicity levels. I have stopped having to take antacids on a daily basis and have stopped getting sinus infections and bronchitis—after getting them every year for almost twenty years. I have completed over twenty triathlons, including Ironman Distance triathlons. I have experienced tremendous energy, and, in fact, have not been sick for years—besides the occasional onsets of fatigue and soreness after multiple sessions of extreme exercise which quickly disappear as a result of my body's ability to recover quickly from this acidic and inflammatory state.

The point to realize is that you can be what society labels as successful, healthy, and fit and not actually be that way at all. It wasn't until I achieved great health that I realized exactly what great health was and how it was truly different from average health. As I will explain in more detail later, before I achieved extreme health, I went to a top high school in Brooklyn, New York; I graduated in the top five of my platoon at Parris Island Marine Corps boot camp, and I was valedictorian at my first college and magna cum laud at my graduate school. I also worked in elite accounting firms; became a CPA, a real estate agent, a multiple franchise owner, an options trader, and an Internet entrepreneur; ran in the New York City Marathon; and completed an Ironman triathlon. Many would see these accomplishments as very successful. I always looked at it as just doing something I had set my mind to do and that there was no stopping me. I always knew there were those who achieved so much more on paper. Maybe they were even truly happy and successful and rich and giving back to society and contributing to the world—instead of just selfishly sucking up all its resources and not serving in a way that benefited at least a few people. I didn't feel that way. I felt I could do more and needed to take myself to a place deep down within that made me feel is if I had achieved that balance and that, in fact, I had taken back control of my life. I had decided I wanted to become that Ironman triathlete and needed to go through the steps, both mentally and physically, of taking control of my life back. For me, the Ironman gave me a sense of purpose. It is a different reason to get up every morning and a great motivator. Part of this story describes that incredible journey also and the role that superfoods had in that journey.

I decided upon having my superfood awakening that I needed to control my own thoughts and to reeducate my beliefs. It is great to learn from other people's experiences and mistakes, but you have to align your consciousness with what instinctually feels right for you. This is true for whom you align yourself with emotionally, the occupation you choose, and—by far the most important—being what you put in your mouth to eat. As I tell my story, I want to impress upon you that although your past experiences may by slightly different, may not seem as dramatic, or may be on the opposite end of the spectrum and be extremely more dramatic or even traumatic, the goal is to take us from how we are thinking and eating to a place where our thinking and eating support us, help us change bad habits, and don't hinder us.

Chapter Two – The Sprouts
of our childhood

At eight years old, I observed a lot of drinking and drugging in my neighborhood. I was able to sneak a can of beer once in a while from the fridge and drink it in my basement. I had to see what all the excitement about partying was all about. After all, I lived in a neighborhood where most everyone walked around with a small brown bag with a beer can in it. Back then, life was as great as an eight-year-old knew it could be. You don't know what is going on outside of a few blocks from your house when you grow up in the city. As a kid growing up in Brooklyn, you primarily know of the kids who live on your street, where the bullies live who will knock you in the head on the way to school, and where the local candy store is.

My parents separated when I was around ten, and my mom did everything she could to raise six kids—which then grew to be nine kids. I was the second oldest and was somewhat shy as a kid. I was very involved with street sports and games. My diet at the time was based on the best we could afford, which at the time was all I really cared for. I don't think the concept of superfoods was around in the 1970s, and if it was, it was not known to my parents or to any other parents that I knew. The standard diet was meat, potatoes, and vegetables, with an occasional pizza. We were on public assistance, as were many in my neighborhood, so extras didn't come that often. I never felt deprived. You don't know what you don't know as a child. Growing up in Brooklyn is a great experience, but it can certainly have its disadvantages. I live in the suburbs now, and the air quality is much better, as are the scenery and the calmness in the air. In Brooklyn, you are truly living in an asphalt jungle of traffic, smog, and what seems like constant danger at times from traffic conditions, wandering homeless people and addicts. At least as you get older you are always more cautious as you walk in the street at night. One of the high schools I went to was considered one of the best in New York City. My grades were always fantastic in school, and I took the test you needed to take to get into—and was able to get into—this above-average high school.

You see, intelligence doesn't always equate to common sense, and vice versa. Being an A student doesn't guarantee a life of being prosperous, being spiritual, and having great health. If there is anything that I learned, it is that those who truly have the gift of academic intelligence—or even street-smart intelligence—have to be careful not to outsmart themselves. You indeed could be your own worst enemy. You begin to overanalyze every situation in your career, in a relationship and with your health. You need to get out of this form of neurosis and get out of your head and into your heart. When you get into your heart and how you feel about something, you make decisions that will serve you better. I remember getting into fights and trying to think of every move that I learned. Should I do a roundhouse kick at this point or a jab followed by an elbow? In reality, most fights end in less than twelve seconds, and too much thinking could leave you dead. I was knocked out once as I stood there trying to decide if I would hit the person with my right or my left first.

The point is that there isn't a clear-cut answer to life when it comes to making the right decisions, and if you overanalyze your life, you may never get to a satisfying destination. For me, this destination has been feeling awesome every day. When you feel awesome every day, you have self-esteem and you feel happy. Isn't that the place we all are trying to get to? How many of us use drugs, alcohol, food and relationships to get to that place? When I was fifteen years old, alcohol was leading me to other things that could have led me down a much worse path than I was already following. One day, someone handed me a needle, and some higher power was definitely on my side. For once, I thought rationally and said no. I don't know why, to this day, that I said no, because I was in a car with three others who were smoking cocaine and shooting heroin, but I was able to hold off the peer pressure.

There are many reasons which I have looked at which were responsible for that decision. My mom was always hard on us to do our homework and get home on time. While I was living in a neighborhood where many were high school dropouts, alcoholics, or drug addicts, the discipline that was instilled in me probably saved my life—because deep down inside, I knew if I took that hit of heroin, I would probably pass out and not be able to go home. I knew that I would be dropping out of school like everyone else, because I had already cut out of school for close to a whole year. Changes surely had to be made quickly if I was going to resurrect myself.

I watched *First Blood* with Sylvester Stallone almost daily. He didn't do drugs. He was a highly trained special forces soldier who didn't like the way society was treating him after he served his country. I wanted to be like Rambo. I wanted to serve my country. I wanted to be tough. I heard of all those swat team guys, the cage fighters, undercover CIA, mercenaries, delta force. Why couldn't I do something like that? I thought if I could be like Rambo, I would satisfy my need for respect, adventure, and esteem more than doing that needle of heroin. I remember walking up to the recruiting station on a Sunday morning in September of 1982 on a cloudy day, with my long hair, cutoff jean jacket, and a pack of cigarettes in my pocket, and I was all set to join the special forces. I had no idea what the training was like, but I had enough confidence in myself to be able to do anything. I got that from my mom, because she always said I could do anything I put my mind to, and I proved that to myself in sports and in school.

I was always in the top 5 percent or better in everything I did. When I walked into the recruiting station, I remember walking over to the army office and putting my hands up to the window so I could see in. Someone put his hand on my shoulder and said, "Can I help you, son?" I turned around in a fighting stance instinctually, to be greeted by the largest man I had ever seen in my life. It was a marine with summer dress blues. I told him I was looking to join the Green Berets, and he looked at me in a way that I knew he hadn't taken me seriously. He said, "Not smoking these," as he took the cigarette pack out of my jean jacket. I totally forgot they were in there and was really embarrassed. What right did I have as a cigarette smoking, alcoholic teenager with long hair to join the Green Berets—never mind the marines? At the time, I didn't even know what the marines were. My thoughts of marines were guys who got out of the water and killed everyone in sight with a bayonet in their mouth. He grabbed me by the shoulder and said, "Come in here and look at this boy." I watched a truly inspiring marine corps recruit video, and the staff sergeant said to me that I really didn't want to go into the Green Berets. He said that first of all, I would have to go through regular army boot camp—and he said it was nothing like the marines and that only a few select army guys got selected to be Green Berets. He said that, based on the way I looked, I wouldn't be one of them. He said that I probably wouldn't even be able to get into the marines, never mind the army elite forces. Excuse me! No one tells me that I can't do something. I was the smartest in my class, and I could hit a Spalding and a "pinky" farther than any kid in the neighborhood. He went on to tell me that the marines had their own version of special forces called force recon and also had airborne units. Now I was interested. I wanted to be airborne. I wanted to get off the streets. I wanted to be the marine version of Rambo. Now, for all the veterans who are reading this and who may even have had special forces training in either the army, navy, air force, or marines, at that moment I had no idea what I was in for, and I'm sure you didn't either before you went in. Not to mention that I was only seventeen years old and completely out of shape.

The recruiter needed to determine what my academic status was in high school. They were only accepting high school graduates. Oh, no! I had skipped school for a whole year. You see—getting back to outsmarting ourselves—we have the capability of being our own worst enemies. The power of our thoughts will control our behavior and our health. The substances I was putting into my body whether it be junk food or cigarette smoke or alcohol, were not helping me think clearly. I could have easily gotten a scholarship to one of the best colleges in America if I had applied myself, or I could have been the best jewel thief in America. We all have choices to make that will shape our destiny. We need to control our own destiny, or something (or someone) else will. That reminds me of a great quote by Jim Rohn: "If you don't design your own life plan, chances are you'll fall into someone else's plan. And guess what they have planned for you? Not much."

The recruiter told me that I had so many credits that despite skipping the entire eleventh grade, I could still graduate on time if I took just two extra classes. This made me proud. I felt I was being given a second chance. I would have to admit to experimenting with marijuana. After all, the recruiter had asked me straight out and I wasn't going to lie about it. Integrity had always been important to me. Despite being somewhat of a juvenile delinquent, I had always felt the value of telling the truth. I was lucky enough to not get caught with anything I had done as a teenager, except once, and that was when I was tracked down by a detective for harassing his mom on a corner we were partying on. He went on to beat my head into the concrete and picked me up over his head and threw me. I deserved it. I didn't throw any punches and just let him do to me what I had done to his mom—which was humiliate her by destroying the front of her house and disturb her by constant loitering outside the house with friends. I had a choice to get arrested or take a beating. I took the beating.

Chapter Three – The Marines

I never went to high school graduation. My first day of boot camp was the same day as graduation. It was the summer of 1983 and it was one of the hottest I could remember. I ended up in third brigade, which had a reputation of being the toughest on the island. That was fine with me. I never took the easy road to anything I ever did. My drill instructors seemed to never stop yelling the first three weeks. There was always one of them taking a turn at getting in our face. They wanted to get rid of all the weak recruits who went into the marines to get out of some trouble they were in, or for the money, or to get out of their houses and away from their parents. They only wanted marines. I had to make my own decision early on. I knew I had gone in to find a new life for myself—away from the life that would inevitably end up in a prison or a casket. After all, that's where all my friends were. It wasn't going to be a piece of cake. However, I never thought it was not doable. In a way, I would laugh inside as I was being yelled at. There were times when your heart was racing at maximum pumps per minute and you were being yelled at by three drill instructors at once and being pushed even further physically. It is at these moments that the weak will break down. Even the toughest will feel the emotions inside but somehow find a way to endure the pain, the emotions, the anger, the confusion, and the mystery of every second that lay in front of you. But isn't that what combat would be like? That's what we were being taught. They wanted to take it as close to the realities of combat as possible. I don't know whether that was possible, but they sure had to try. I ended up a squad leader after like the third or fourth week into boot camp. I could march well and I was disciplined. I'm not sure the drill instructors liked me at all.

The Brooklyn attitude surely rubbed off of me. In fact, all the guys they put in my squad were city boys. I suppose they figured they would keep all the potential troublemakers in one place where we could be watched. We ended up having a great squad and I was proud of all of them—everyone that made it through those thirteen weeks in 90 degree heat plus humidity, all thirty-nine of us that survived from the original seventy-two. I shot expert with the rifle and would go on to shoot expert five more times while in the corps. When I was getting out of the marine corps, in fact, I was asked if I had an interest in the marine corps rifle team or sniper school, but I didn't have any interest in reenlisting at the time. I would regret that later as I watched my unit go to combat a few times in the years that followed.

You never really want to go to combat, but you can't help but want to use your training and be with your fellow marines. My experiences in the marine corps led me to many places, including Korea, Thailand, Cuba, Puerto Rico, Spain, Turkey, and Okinawa. I was told when I enlisted that in order to get into force recon, I would have to go through marine infantry. I decided to take my chances with an enlistment bonus program that would pay me a three-thousand-dollar bonus, but I would have to take the chance of ending up in an MOS (military occupational specialty) that may not have been my ideal choice. Unfortunately, I ended up in artillery as a forward observer at first. We were the guys who went ahead and set up an observation post close to enemy territory so we could map out targets of opportunity. At first I thought I would hate the job, but in my typical fashion, if I was going to do something, I was going to be the best at it. And I was.

I graduated near the top of my classes and I received meritorious commendations for my work while under general inspections. I had been assigned overseas during my first year, and some of my Brooklyn ways were coming back. I started to drink heavily again. In fact, before I went to Okinawa, Japan, a gunnery sergeant who was one of the marine corps poster boys and who was highly decorated and respected predicted that I wouldn't even come back from Okinawa. He predicted I would die over there. He was wrong. I did, however, get really depressed, and it seemed like I still had an eternity left in the marines. I wasn't eating the best foods. I would eat whatever was being served in the chow hall or what was being served out in town at food stands. I had no idea what I was eating most of the time. I was highly acidic, always hung over, and always dehydrated.

Almost daily, I would come in at 4:00 AM and have to go on a four-mile run at 4:30 AM. I would sneak in an hour or two nap at lunchtime to sober up, and after evening formation I headed out to town again with one of many friends I had made, including one who was from New Jersey. He had spent time in an airborne unit before going to Okinawa. He would talk for hours about his experiences, and I looked up to him as a leader and a friend. I so wanted to have done what he did. He left the island about a week before I did. When I got my orders to go back to the States, I was in shock. I was headed to the same elite airborne unit that he was in before he came to Okinawa. I already knew everything about the unit. I knew that they were commanded by a special operations three-star general and were sent on special advance party deployments to places of hostility. I knew they had an exercise program that was more rigorous than most units in the military. Yikes! Was this really happening? Just as in September of 1982 when I first joined the marines and had nine months to get myself in shape for boot camp, I had about five weeks before I had to check in with my unit.

It was now October of 1985 and I was twenty years old and about to check into an airborne unit and get what I had always asked for. Even though I had already been in the marines for two and a half years, I was going to be treated like I was in boot camp again. When I checked into the unit, I was immediately greeted by another highly decorated veteran gunnery sergeant, and he didn't want any part of me—who I was, where I was coming from, or where I thought I wanted to go. This experience was just like boot camp, where you had no idea what you were doing or why you were there. You just knew deep down you were in deep shit and weren't going to quit no matter what. He didn't like the way I talked, the way I was dressed, my haircut, or my record book. For all intents and purposes, I was a shit bird. I had gotten in trouble in Okinawa for telling a corporal to f—— off. In this unit, there was none of that. It was yes, Corporal; no, Corporal…yes, Sergeant; no, Sergeant. Discipline, integrity, and honor were the name of the game, and if you didn't want to be the best, you weren't welcome. I did want to be the best, but I wasn't welcome anyway—at least not yet.

I was sent to get a haircut three times before it was acceptable to the "gunny." I had to press my uniform, shine my boots, stand at attention like I was two inches taller than I really was, and scream as loud as I could in the push-up position that I was sure I wanted to be there because they were going to be keeping a real close eye on Will Power. I was sent down to third brigade. This was the leg brigade—the brigade you went to when you hadn't qualified yet for jump school. The brigade where you had to learn how to call in air strikes and naval gunfire, do fifty push-ups in less than two minutes, eighty sit-ups in less than two minutes, and ten dead-hang pull-ups and four miles in less than twenty-eight minutes. This was tough for me. I was still over two hundred pounds from the drink fest in Okinawa.

When I walked by the third brigade office, they wanted to know who the hell I was and why I was standing on their handprints. I looked down, and indeed I was standing on their handprints. The problem was my hands were not on them. I was in the push-up position doing push-ups for what seemed like an entire morning. You couldn't walk in the office without doing push-ups first. I remind you that this was the regular marine corps. Boot camp had been two and a half years ago and was long over, so I thought. They told me right up front they were not going to have any attitude from me and that I probably wasn't going to make it. Of course, I was in survival instinct mode. Who the hell did they think they were talking to? I had already been through more in my life than most people, and I wasn't going to let some cowboys tell me I couldn't do anything. You want me to run twenty-two miles with a log on my shoulder, then let's go. I may not make it a mile, but I'm in. Let's do it.

Over the course of the next three months or so, I would prove to them what I was all about. I was the only one ever in the unit's history to score one hundred on their written test, and I had gotten my four-mile time down from thirty-six minutes to fewer than twenty-seven. I was chosen to go to jump school finally in January of 1986 in front of several peers who had gotten to third brigade before me. I was transformed once again. My diet, however, had not changed. I was still eating badly. Although I had quit alcohol, I was still eating unconsciously. One of the ideals I would learn was that you have to eat consciously to get the full effect of extreme health. To get the benefits of being totally present and grounded, you need to have both the right foods and the right intentions of the foods' purpose and why you are eating.

I ended up being meritoriously promoted to corporal in this unit and finally fulfilled a dream of being an elite, airborne, special operations marine. I had the opportunity to jump twenty-three times out of planes and helicopters; to hang from helicopters and be inserted into tree lines, airports, the ocean and to jump at night; to go through survival training, chemical warfare training, and rifle and pistol coach school; and to get in great physical shape. I also would have never gone to college if it hadn't been for my roommate, who ended up signing me up for college even after enduring my never ending reluctance. I had always said I would never go to college. It just wasn't in my family history and it was just never thought of as something I would do—until two months before I got out of the marines, when my roommate said with a certain satire that he would feel it was his fault if I ended up dead on a street corner in Brooklyn if he didn't sign me up for college. I would do the same for one of my brothers a year later and would also encourage another brother to go into the marines when he was twenty-five and seemed to be at a crossroads in his life.

Chapter Four – College and Corporate America

I ended up going to a college in Long Island, New York, and I joined the cross-country team. When I was in the marines, we had often gone on thirteen to fifteen-mile runs, and I felt the cross-country team was something I should give a try. I had no idea what cross-country even was. Did it mean to run across the country? I figured I would run across the countryside like I did in the marines, but without the combat gear and logs. I was in for another awakening of a different sort. I once again showed up with a pack of cigarettes in my sleeve and told the coach I wanted to join. I said I had just run eight miles that day, and even though I had smoked a little over the summer, I was going to give it up for good. He looked at me skeptically. I was 203 pounds and the rest of the team was 140 pounds. "No worries," I said as he mentioned they were doing ten miles easy that day. They went out at about a seven-thirty- to eight-minute-mile pace, and for me it was like a race from the start. They occasionally would turn around to see if I was still alive but were way ahead of me on this so-called "easy" day. My coach asked me how I felt afterwards, but I couldn't answer. I just said, "See you tomorrow," in typical Will Power fashion. If you haven't yet seen the trend, my whole life has been a trend of ups and downs—a roller coaster life of bad food addictions, accomplishments, proving to myself I could overcome all odds against me, and always seeking fulfillment.

That first day of practice was the beginning of two of the greatest years of my life. Those first two years of running cross-country and track with that team kept me inspired for years to come and still to this day I am inspired from the memories of running in elite events at Harvard and Yale University. Looking back on that first day, when they thought they would never see me again, until my last practice with them was filled with great memories. They would see me go on to win "most improved athlete," become valedictorian in my curriculum, sing cadences to them while we were on our runs, and always be there to motivate them. I went on to another four-year university in New York, because I had a scholarship to go into their accounting program. Another key mentor in my life was an accounting professor, who also had his masters in computer science. He was one of the only professors on the Internet in the school, and he said anyone that could get the grades that I got on his test should become a CPA (like he was). So I did. Mostly at the time because I knew I could.

I knew this school had a great accounting program, and I knew they had a cross-country and track team. I would get a small track scholarship and a huge academic scholarship, which paid for most of my expenses. For the remainder of the cost, I would take out student loans, work full time, and pay them off over ten years. I had the same experiences at this school as I had in the two-year college. We went to track meets almost every weekend. I don't know how I would have gotten through the rigorous MBA program I was in without being on the team. Even though it added to the amount of hours of work, it helped balance out the crazy academic schedule. The same habits my mom helped me develop in grammar school carried on to college, and it was seldom that I didn't get an A. I also was able to get down to 175 pounds and be good enough to feel competitive at the meets which we participated in. My five-mile cross-country time got down to near thirty minutes from thirty-eight minutes in my first race. These were some of the toughest courses in the northeast, at Sunken Meadow State Park in Long Island and Van Cortland Park in the Bronx.

A guy of my size had no business in the track-and-field business. I was actually so good at other sports like softball that I don't know why I didn't bother trying out for the baseball team. It was one of those things where the endurance required of being a marine carried over in my mentality, and when I was standing in front of the school bulletin board in August of 1987 and I was looking over all the sport team tryouts, the first ones to jump out at me were soccer and cross-country. I felt I had no business trying out for baseball. I wasn't on a Little League team for my whole life like others. Yes, I hit home run after home run on the streets down at the school, but that was with all my bully friends—not on a real team with a coach and uniforms. I almost felt like I just didn't belong there. I had played soccer in the marines, and I played when I was about ten through thirteen as a kid in Brooklyn. I was coached by my boss in the store I worked in, who was semi-professional.

At my first soccer practice in college, I pulled a hamstring and was embarrassed and never went back. I was originally going to do both sports, but the next day was that first cross-country practice, which made me realize that I needed to focus on just the cross-country. I sometimes wish I had gone back to that second soccer practice. As the years went by in college, I continued to make great friends and have great roommates. Every experience taught me something, and I always had the chance to inspire others with my experiences. I ate chef salads seemingly every day. I thought they were healthy because they had lettuce and meat in them. My life seemed to have taken shape in small blocks of experiences.

I would begin to learn that I wasn't of a typical mold. I certainly had a rough childhood compared to most, and I was running on my own intuitions, which were shaded with addictions and were perhaps misguided at times. I always felt like I was moving forward, though. I had gotten great grades and began to study for the CPA exam like I had committed to do. I interviewed with all six of the Big 6 public accounting firms and got three offers. I accepted one of them and went on to pass each part of the CPA exam on the first try with lots of room to spare. In fact, I over-studied. It was a nineteen and a half–hour exam in total at the time, and I simply blew it away. Where did it get me?

Well, you set out to achieve something and there is some satisfaction in that; but I spent so much time in my life to meet that goal, and the payoff wasn't as great as I anticipated, because I just didn't put the efforts into capitalizing on that career. People like me figure out real fast whether something is serving you in a healthy and supportive way or in an unhealthy and unsupportive way. Since I had started to drink again after staying away from it for close to seven years, I knew something wasn't working. I left public accounting and took on a corporate accounting job. The best thing to happen to me while I was in public accounting was that I met my wife. We hit it off right from the start, and I knew I wanted to marry her the day she said she would always cherish the ground I walked on. And she has. I would move into a small five-million-dollar company for a couple of years until I realized there might have been something going on there that wasn't in the highest of integrity. I was always a man of integrity. That's just the way I always felt most comfortable being.

I bought into a retail store franchise and pretty much put everything I owned on the line. I wanted out of corporate America so bad, and I had great credit and easily got loans for the startup capital. At around the same time, I made a move to a small software company. This was more my style. It was laid back, and I could learn to write software programs and still use my accounting and business background to understand clients' operations and systems. I ended up staying at this company almost ten years in a full- or part-time capacity; however, I left when I decided to spend full time on my retail and Internet businesses. During this ten-year period—while I was married, working for the software company, becoming a dad, buying my first and second houses, and then becoming my own version of an entrepreneur—I was sort of on cruise control.

Chapter Five – The Awakening Begins

The awakening had not yet happened. There were great moments in my life—like having my first child, then my second, completing the NYC marathon, and getting my name on a book I coauthored. I was eating better and was not drinking heavily, and I certainly was keeping myself in shape running whenever I could by entering road races. There was something missing, and I started to search for it by going to conferences and seeing great peak performance coaches speak, like Anthony Robbins, T. Harv Ecker, Mark Victor Hansen, Les Brown, Robert Kiyosaki, and Jack Canfield. Awakenings do not happen overnight, although it seems to have taken a lifetime of experiences to believe that I had one. When everything you have ever done comes together, and you start to define your purpose and your passions begin to unfold, it is then that the awakening is complete. I believe for some people that awakening can happen in an instant. It is in that one "aha" moment that it all comes together.

I would say that this chapter of my life started in January 2007, when I was at a conference which was meant to help you figure out your life direction. You go through a series of exercises, like writing your own eulogy, drawing out your mission and visions for your life, etc. A common theme that kept coming up for me was completing an Ironman triathlon. I hadn't even done a triathlon or biathlon yet in my life. I had years of road, track, and cross-country experience, with lots of memories, but those experiences led me to many injuries which had put doubts in my mind as to my ability to continue as an endurance athlete. In the year 2000, when I was at one of my heavy stages, I decided to lose some weight and get back into running. For the previous seven years, corporate America had taken its toll on my health. After all, I allowed it to. All the decisions were mine—where I worked and who I hung out with. I had determined my own destiny. It can be said that the five people you hang around with the most will determine your health and your net worth.

Everything I ate and drank was my own choice. Every job I took was my own choice. I could have gone into the woods and lived off the land and my own garden, or I could have taken a corporate high-stress job and eaten fast food every day, or somewhere in between. Balance is the key for a life where everything seems normal. However, sometimes greatness is hard to achieve with balance. Michael Phelps does not have what most would consider balance. He swims five hours a day, eats eight to ten thousand calories, and sleeps in between. This is one end of the balance spectrum that most people would not be able to handle, which is why most are not the best Olympians ever. Therefore, even balance comes down to making choices. When we are younger, we seem to be able to handle less balance, to one extreme or the other. Our bodies are detoxifying better, so it doesn't seem as important to eat great.

I received a card in the mail from Team in Training in early 2000, inviting me to raise money for the Leukemia & Lymphoma Society in return for training me for a marathon. I had completed a marathon twelve years earlier in New York, when I was in phenomenal shape and at a weight of 169 pounds. I had grown to about 210 pounds and wanted to get down to about 200. My addictive behavior took over, and it seemed that every week I was entering races. I ran twenty-six races that year, but the marathon gave me a serious IT band injury that would bother me for years to come. I didn't know how to treat my body with anything but antibiotics when I got sick. All the doctors would say was to drink more fluids and to take these pills. This went on for seven years, and all the doctors would say was that some people weren't meant to be runners and I should stop and take on some other form of exercise.

Running was all I knew, and I was stubborn and didn't want to stop. Every time I ran, I would make it about two miles and my IT band would start hurting. So you can imagine that when I was at that life directions conference thinking about doing my first Ironman within five years, I was slightly kidding myself. Deep down, I couldn't help but think I was seriously injured back in 2000 and I probably tore a muscle that never healed right. I signed up for another course in February of 2007 called "extreme health."

This conference was four days of all day and night intense back-to-back seminars with exercise sessions built in. We also did a 10K. I hadn't run a full 6.2 miles in a few years. However, I had been sober for a month and had started to become more alkaline. I had been eating what I thought was right and stretching quite a bit to stay flexible. I was doing other exercises to increase strength in the legs and core muscles. I was able to finish in the top ten out of a few hundred that ran the course. It wasn't a race, but more of a fun run, yet I still wanted to run the whole way without stopping. I had run under thirty-eight minutes for the same distance in a road race when I was in college, and that image of me sprinting to the finish always crosses my mind when I do a 10K. Even if I only do a 10K in an hour, I feel the same thrill as I did back when I was younger and faster.

I did run the whole way during that 10K at the conference, and it felt great to not feel as injured as I had previously. There was a transformation taking place in my body just from my being sober and eating right for one month. This is an important concept for people working on improving their health. The body can heal itself when it is given the chance. It needs the right fuel. I felt that a higher power was telling me something at this conference. The speakers at this conference talked about everything from herbs to sleeping better. There were demonstrations of various health and fitness tools; there were talks about the skin and dieting in general. Nothing affected me as much as when David Wolfe walked on the stage with his poncho on. He looked at the crowd and wanted to dedicate his talk to all the organic farmers who were trying to make a difference in the world. This was the talk I had been waiting for all my life. I knew it was on organic foods, but I had no idea the impact it would make on my entire thought process about life and so eloquently weave together years of learning of what I had taught myself about nutrition. I was about to experience what I earlier called a superfood awakening. It's similar to that "aha" moment. It's when every light bulb in your entire system turns on at the same time. It took just a few Kirlian images on the screen and a few sentences related to how important it was to eat *live* food. How could I go forty years without knowing this? I had instincts that gave me clues over the years. When I ate a burned piece of meat, for instance, I would say to myself, *This just doesn't seem right. How could this be good for you? It looks like cancer. It's dark, black, cooked, and dead.* I would eat it anyway.

I also felt the same way about microwave ovens. Something inside me knew it was wrong. It just doesn't make sense to see a light for one minute and a loud buzzing sound which bubbles the outer edges of the food but leaves other parts cold. I would say to friends that someday wouldn't it be funny if they found out microwave ovens were the cause of cancer. Little did I know that, as I became more involved with my own health, I would discover that some countries actually ban the use of microwave ovens because their testing indicates that the ovens do play a role in causing certain types of cancer.

As David Wolfe spoke about raw foods and superfoods, it was as if everything I had learned or instinctually believed since I was sixteen years old was brought together at one moment. It was as if I immediately knew what to do to heal myself and to get to a point where I had the best health ever.

The rest of this book is going to cover a lifetime of learning that I have experienced in regards to nutrition and how the notion of eating raw, organic, living, plant-based superfoods and introducing other holistic health practices into your life will completely stack the odds in your favor for living a long, healthy life. I will go over the specific foods that I eat and how they helped me overcome years of chronic bronchitis, and how I trained for and successfully completed my first Ironman as a Clydesdale athlete (over two-hundred-pound athlete).

Diets do not work if you are trying to change a habit. A diet is designed to make you follow a specific "do this; don't do that" format. Most people have problems with that whole concept habitually. Ever since we were kids, we were always told, "Don't do this" or "Don't do that." And what did we do? We did it anyway. It's very difficult to expect someone to stick with a diet that does not give them a superfood awakening moment like I had in February 2007. When you have the superfood awakening—or sometimes I call it an organic awakening—moment, you are giving yourself permission to change. You are giving yourself permission to not do or to do something. That is a huge difference in whether you are going to be successful at something.

Making the decision to add more living foods to your body is not a diet decision. It is a decision that you are willing to do what it takes to feel good. Most people know instinctually what they need to do. Others believe that they are doing a good job, but once they get the critical missing information and are willing to work with it, they could take their health to a whole new level. There are many diets out there that appear to work for some people. In fact, some work for some people and some appear to work for others at least at first, because at a minimum the diet they are following is much better than anything else they were doing up to that point. So if someone starts to feel good after a couple of weeks, they spread the word and that diet becomes popular. Changing a lifestyle does not become as popular, because the change seems more radical. "You mean I can't eat eggplant parmigiana anymore because it has trans fats in the fried oil?" Anytime there is a set of rules around a diet, it becomes harder to follow. That's why the concept of *adding* foods into your existing food intake is a better path. The good food starts to crowd out the bad. I learned this from David Wolfe and found it to be a powerful concept.

I have always been one to want a complete picture of everything that I need to do. Then I can make a conscious choice of what to do, knowing it is my own fault if I choose to take a different path. For instance, we all know what the speed limit is on the roads where we drive. This is good information, just like it is good information for someone to say it is healthy to eat more spices. But what if you had more information that could help you make an even better decision? Many people speed despite knowing what the speed limit is. What if they knew what the consequences were of going five miles an hour over the limit, or ten or even twenty? What if they knew they could lose their license if they went over twenty-five miles an hour over the speed limit? Then if they went over twenty-five miles an hour over the limit, they would be consciously disobeying the law regardless of the known consequences. When someone is making a conscious decision, there isn't much you can do to change them. Some people actually tell me they just don't give a damn. If you don't like it, then get out of their way. Same goes for people who know something is bad for them and say, "Who cares? You're not going to live forever anyway." They are consciously eating badly. I worry more about the people who are unknowingly and unconsciously eating badly.

For instance, what if instead of someone saying you should eat more spices, he says that if you eat more turmeric, you may decrease your chances of getting certain cancers, that turmeric can be anti-inflammatory and is supposed to be a superior antioxidant because recent studies have shown this to be true? Or what if someone said that once they stopped drinking and eating dairy products, a lifetime of ear infections went away or they stopped getting bronchitis every year or they were able to lose weight for the first time in years? Would that make someone say, "Wait a minute. I thought we needed to drink milk to get calcium for our strong bones. That's what all the advertisements say." I know there are people who are very one-dimensional in their thinking. Something they learned twenty years ago is cemented into their thinking, and it would take the president of the United States banning milk on public television for them to stop drinking it. I think this is a tragedy in today's society, because we need to get to a point where we take control of our own health and take the control away from the media, the doctors, the advertisements, and the old-school ancestors.

The health field is continually evolving, and new information is being discovered all the time. This information doesn't always get to us in an efficient way. It may even be blocked and criticized by groups whose profits would be affected by the release of the information. I am not a doctor, but I do not have to be one to share what my own body has done for me. Yes, my own body healed itself. Is that old news? There were no drugs thousands of years ago. When you look at the life span of people thousands of years ago, it does not compare to today on average. However, this is another area where you need to use common sense. People were malnourished without the knowledge of essential minerals and vitamins that were needed. People were exposed to diseases that they were not aware of how to avoid; people were constantly just killing each other over everything from land to a handful of beans. It isn't drugs that have extended our life span in my opinion—it is higher-quality living and awareness of how to avoid sickness. There is only one person that can cure anything in this world in my opinion, and that is your own body. There is nothing more powerful than your immune system running on all its cylinders. Think about the possibilities of having the most awesome health ever. Imagine being able to always have energy and being able to fight off sickness before it takes control of you and makes you reach for drugs and medicines. I have lived that life for close to two years, despite training for an Ironman triathlon and despite being told I shouldn't run anymore. Does that qualify me to share with you my experiences? I think it does. In fact, I feel it's my duty to share my experiences in the hope that you will be turned on to the possibilities.

In February of 2007, I experienced my first piece of real chocolate. I hadn't realized I had never had real chocolate before. I hadn't realized that most chocolate bars were processed versions of the real thing. They contained dairy products and sugars. They contained guarana and kola nut, which increased the caffeine amounts. They were roasted and cooked, and therefore the life force energy I spoke of as being the most important nutritional factor for me was zapped out of them. The chocolate I was introduced to was Sacred Heart chocolate and raw cacao beans. The raw cacao bean looks like an almond and contains 100 percent raw chocolate. This cacao bean is the single greatest source of antioxidants on the planet. This includes blueberries, mangosteen, acai berry juice, and grapes. Cacao is also one of the greatest sources of magnesium and vitamin C, as well as a great source of iron. Cacao is also a food for the heart. Magnesium is critical for proper heart function, and women have intuitively known this for years. Cacao is also a great weight loss food because it seems to be so rich in minerals that it turns off food cravings, which I believe are really mineral or thirst cravings. When your body craves food, it is craving the minerals in the food. Cacao is also rich in chromium, which helps control blood sugar levels. Most of society seems to have trouble with blood sugar.

I am a vegetarian, and more than 70 percent of what I eat is raw, plant-based, and organic. What that means to me is that I choose not to eat red meats and focus on plant-based foods. There are several stages of vegetarianism. I started off first with eating less barbecued food. I then went to eating less food that was cooked in the oven. I then went to not eating red meat at all. I then started to minimize my intake of dairy products, chicken, turkey, and fish to about once a month. I started to eat organic eggs only once a week, then once every two weeks, instead of three times a week. This progression happened naturally for me. In other words, the more good superfoods I added to my diet, the more they would crowd out the other foods. It was easy to cut back on these foods, because I didn't want them anymore. If I did want them, then I would have eaten them. However, the combination of my knowledge of other foods which were better for me took over any cravings I had for the animal foods. In fact, it isn't a surprise to me that something that grows in nature is healthier for me than something that comes from a dead animal. That is common sense for me. All living creatures eat what grows. I am not one to believe that we need meat from animals to survive, because the animals themselves survive off of foods from nature. Even fish, which we are told are essential for our diets so we can get the omega-3 fatty acids, are just not needed. Big fish eat smaller fish, which eat even smaller fish. Well, guess what the smallest fish are eating. They are eating plants and algae off the ocean floor.

In fact, marine phytoplankton, which scientists say were the start of life on earth a few billion years ago, are the food source of some of the largest sharks and whales in the world, some of which live to over 150 years old. The nutrient profile of phytoplankton is off the charts. They contain most, if not all, of the vitamins and minerals known to man, as well as all the amino acids. There have been many documented cases of people who have healed themselves much quicker with phytoplankton. Phytoplankton even contain those omega-3's, that fish have—which makes sense, since the fish are eating the phytoplankton. My thought process is, Why process all these great foods through fish and animals when we could go straight to the source the animals are getting them from?

Chapter Six – Ironman Dreams

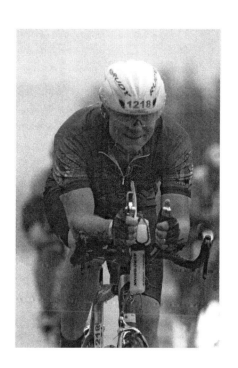

When I came to the conclusion that with foods I could possibly heal my body from a lifetime of injuries, I realized that my dream of becoming an Ironman triathlete could be a reality. If Michael Phelps could become the best athlete in the world while eating out at restaurants and eating tons of cooked foods, then I could become an Ironman despite my size and health by taking my diet to the highest of levels. Nutrition obviously isn't the only thing that makes an athlete great. There are genetic factors in the athlete's shape and size, as well as the athlete's ability to generate ATP (Adenosine-5'-triphosphate), utilize their potential VO2 levels, fight lactic acid buildup, recover from exercise by controlling inflammation, control oxidative stress, and detoxify the body. ATP is the energy currency within our cells. Some of us genetically are capable of generating higher levels of ATP. Surprisingly enough Phytoplankton actually contains ATP. VO2 is a reflection of the physical fitness of an individual as it measures someone's ability to transport and utilize oxygen. ATP and VO2 are also potentially greater when an athlete is young. As Michael Phelps gets older, there is no doubt that what he did in 2008 in China can be done again if he continues his training but gets on a superfoods diet. The superfoods will just get him to the next level, which at this point is just beating himself. I used the superfood diet to get to my Ironman finish, so I know it works.

As I began to drink my smoothies every morning and eat my organic salads in the afternoons, I would see the weight come off. I joined Team in Training once again in 2007 and signed up to complete my first century ride at Lake Tahoe. One hundred miles on a bike seemed impossible to me at one time in my life. Nothing seems impossible to me anymore. Exercise and diet and passion can get you to your destination faster than anything else. I felt the increase in leg strength would help with what I thought was terrible knees, and I would be able to run again. During the same time period, I also signed up for my first triathlon. It was a Half Ironman in New Hampshire. I hadn't even completed my first sprint triathlon and I was going to do a Half Ironman, which consisted of a 1.2-mile swim, a 56-mile bike ride, and a 13.1-mile run.

There was a problem with this concept. I had never swum more than the length of a round swimming pool. I had never swum in a lake or the ocean more than about twenty feet. And it was my version of what swimming was, which meant my head was out of the water for the most part and I relied on my arm strength to pull me through the water, as my legs would slowly sink as I was swimming. I knew I had to get into a pool and do what I knew I had to do, and that was learn to do what was called "laps." This meant I also had to share lanes with people who already knew how to swim. My first day at the YMCA was somewhat of a major challenge for me. I knew the lifeguard was zoned in on me after I did my first twenty-five yards and jumped up for air. I second-guessed myself. Maybe I should just stick to running. No!! I wasn't going to give up. I will just rest for a minute or two and do another twenty-five yards. This would go on for about a half hour. I did a total of about three hundred yards. The lifeguard was glad to see me get out of the water. He may have actually had to go in the pool and get wet for the first time since he began employment.

After several weeks, I began to get better. I learned what a pull buoy was, and I learned from various swim videos I watched. I had started to go to group swims with Team in Training and learned that I was swimming flat and my head moved too much. I needed to learn how to rotate my shoulders and hips and reach and glide better. I also needed to develop my core muscles so that I could keep my body more on top of the water. I began to be able to swim more than eight hundred yards continuously, and I was eager to sign up for my first sprint triathlon. I wanted to experience the shorter-distance triathlon before I jumped into the Half Ironman. So now, I was simultaneously training for my first sprint triathlon, my first Half Ironman triathlon, and my first century bike ride of one hundred miles—all while rebuilding and detoxifying a lifetime of injuries and illnesses which were previously treated by antibiotics.

My Swim around Lake Placid in 2008

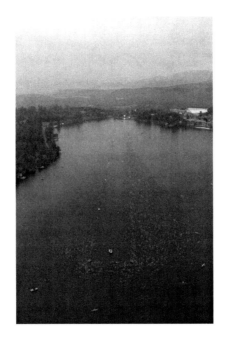

Chapter 7 – How did I cleanse?

Cleansing is an important piece of the equation. David Wolfe had mentioned the word "cleanse" more than once during his lecture, and I wanted to know more about it. My only thought of cleansing was taking a shower. I would later find out that this was actually even more of a reason to cleanse. Our body absorbs water through our skin when we shower, and I did not use a shower filter at home, which meant I was absorbing whatever was in the water. There are so many ways to cleanse different parts of your body. I can share what I did and what I have learned, but everyone at a minimum should walk away with the concept that cleansing is important in helping your body get rid of toxins—especially in the beginning when you are not running on all your cylinders. For instance, if you are overburdening your adrenals, your lymphatic system, and your liver, then your detoxification system is not functioning at 100 percent.

The first thing I started to do was drink clean water. I had studied how important it was to keep our bodies alkaline, to the point where for me it is the single most important factor to our health. In fact, if someone were to ask me what the most important thing to me was in regards to health, I would respond, "to work on getting yourself more alkaline." I believe this, because to do this you need to take a lot of important steps. You need to drink alkaline, ionized water. You need to eat alkaline foods. You need to breathe deeper, fresher air, and you need to keep your stress levels low. If you do all these things, you will certainly change your health for the better. I had also learned that cancer could not survive in an alkaline environment. If that isn't an eye-opener, then what is?

I wouldn't be surprised if some of the most famous people on earth—like Oprah Winfrey or even the president—are not aware of the concept of alkalinity, as important as it is to your overall health. A doctor might be taught this at some point in his education, but it may not be common practice to educate people about it. That's why I educate myself. Who cares more about me than I do? I have sixty trillion cells in my body starving for nutrients every day and trying to get rid of toxins at the same time through my lymphatic system, and it is the food I eat that is going to enable it to do that—not some pill or magic spell. In the end, when you take a pill, aren't you putting something in your mouth at the end of the day anyway. If so, what are the pills made from? Everything comes from the earth as its starting point. So let's keep it there and stop mixing all these compounds together so the process can be patented.

I understand that once people get to a certain point in their health where they are in pretty bad shape, then preventing a disease becomes a moot point. If they already have a disease, then they aren't so willing to rely on foods to get rid of that disease. There is an obvious pressure to go with a drug that seems to have been working for other people, so it must work for them. Maybe the pill does help get rid of some of the symptoms, and I'm sure there are certain diseases that need medication to prevent them from killing you. My point here is to raise awareness in people who have not gotten to the point of needing medication but are trying to prevent themselves from getting to that point, and I think a first step is the water that we drink and the foods that we eat. It is very difficult to get clean water without spending some money and doing some work. You can drive to a local spring and fill up water bottles. This takes time and money, and also, you can not be sure of what is running into those streams that may be toxic. Other than that, spring water is probably one of the best sources of natural water. Another good source is ionized and mineralized distilled water. Distilled water on its own is not so good according to some sources, and not so bad according to some sources. It is pure H_2O which has all of the minerals and bacteria removed through a vaporization process. There seems to be a lot of disagreement in a lot of areas of health, and this is one of them.

Can we dispute that pure water is a bad thing? It is probably a good thing according to my common sense and intuition. Is it true that it leaches out good minerals from your body? There are some that say it does and some that say it doesn't. So maybe a compromise is distilled water which is ionized and has trace minerals added to it. This way, the water becomes more alkaline and you don't have to worry about who is right. We know we need minerals, we know we need water, and having ionized water gives it a charge which some studies have shown also helps the healing process. There are also reverse osmosis triple-filtering systems that you can get for your sink or for your whole house. These systems also attempt to filter out a lot of the contaminants found in tap water. In the end, the water is cleaner but does not contain as many trace minerals. My intuition would tell me that spring water is the best source of water, however. I know most of it is only available in plastic bottles—which bring a whole other set of issues, such as the cost on the environment to get the water in those bottles, as well as the plastic materials which get into the water. I have gone middle of the road on this one. I drink filtered water on occasion, I drink spring water primarily from bottles, and I also add minerals to the water, as well as lemon and goji berries. It is the best that I have been able to do for myself, and I can say that I believe it has contributed to my good health. I realize that toxins are getting into my system from the water I drink, which is another reason I believe in cleansing.

My next method of cleansing is green juices and vegetables. As I began to eat more vegetables, I began to remineralize my body. I think this is important before you start doing harsher cleanses. Your body needs to adjust itself and start to get healthier. Your systems need to start running better. This includes all your systems, such as your digestive system, your immune system, your adrenal system and endocrine system, and your cardiovascular system. Green foods have so many built-in detoxifying properties, such as fiber and antioxidants, as well as phytonutrients. Another major first step in cleansing is to stop putting toxins in your body. In fact, "You are what you don't eat" is just as important as "You are what you eat." Telling people not to eat something is probably the hardest thing anyone can tell someone else. Food can be as powerful as drugs, in my opinion, and people can be just as addicted to a type of food as they are to a bottle of scotch. I speak often on the subject of nutrition, health, wellness, and fitness, to those I come in contact with daily and this has certainly become clear to me. Also, almost everyone wants to lose weight, look better, feel better, have more energy, feel happiness, and just plainly and simply have more fun and enjoy life. However, very few people have the knowledge of how to do it or will listen to any advice, or if they do have good intentions, their actions don't always align with those intentions. They simply have a hard time with change when it comes to lifestyle choices and food choices. After all, as I said earlier, isn't that why most diets fail? Do this, don't do that, eat more of this, eat less of that. It becomes overwhelming and eventually you quit. It's the same concept as for people that want to be rich but aren't willing to make the sacrifices necessary to make the money and keep it in their life.

Whenever I come across people who are not open to taking the appropriate measures to dramatically increase their health, I have to step back. They are often brainwashed by false beliefs and programming from their parents, from advertising and marketing on TV, from fancy labels and packaging, from articles put out by companies trying to make their products look better than what they are, from peer pressure, habitual behavior, etc. After all, isn't wheat good for me? Isn't milk good for me? Most people never even research better choices or whether something truly is good for them. They simply "heard" it was. There are so many better choices in food than what the average person currently consumes. There are better grains (quinoa, amaranth, spelt, millet), better fruits and vegetables (kale, spinach, berries), better snacks (cucumber, peppers, celery), better fats (avocados, olive oil, almonds, flaxseeds) , and better proteins (quinoa, oats, pumpkin and sunflower seeds, nuts, hemp seed, goji berries, and bee pollen). Unless the common people seek out this information, they are doomed to what is offered in local supermarkets. I personally cannot find more than ten items to put in my cart in a typical supermarket, which carries more than fifty thousand items. Why is this? One reason is because the majority of food is not organic, so it is therefore subject to things like pesticides, herbicides, fungicides, hormones, genetic modification, antibiotics, factory processing, preservatives, processed sweeteners, etc.

I understand that not everyone is going to be able to afford a seven-day-a-week organic diet (I sure can't), and not everyone is going to be able to spend countless hours educating themselves in health and wellness. Even health professionals have a hard time keeping up with what is the latest good food, bad food, or super herb, or new anti-aging product. So what can we do to begin to stack the odds in our favor as we slowly move towards better health in a way that works for us? Maybe we can eat one organic meal a week or read one article a week on what is going on in the health industry. The key is moving in the right direction, not a direction that leads to self-destruction. What I am going to suggest is probably one of the biggest steps that someone can take to improve their health for the better—and that is to start reading labels and stop putting certain substances into your body that make it so much harder to lose weight and to absorb nutrients, and to begin to change the tide from bad health to good health.

The first ingredient you absolutely may want to check your cabinets for and eliminate, as well as avoid buying in the future, is partially hydrogenated oils (all forms, such as soybean, canola, cottonseed, palm, vegetable, etc.). That one ingredient is the single ingredient in recent research most closely tied to heart disease. Hydrogenated oils are basically as close to a plastic as you are going to get. They are added to foods to extend the life of the food and for the taste. These oils can cause liver and gall bladder disease; they can cause low birth weights and numerous other problems in kids. The fact is, we have been lied to by the labels on foods simply because we are not ever told the truth.

The second ingredient is high-fructose corn syrup. Combine this with the hydrogenated oils, and you may have one of the most dangerous combinations that you could put in your body. It's your body, and the next time you say "Hmmmm, good" to some cookies from the middle aisle of a grocery store, all I can say is, "Look at the label." It may taste good from the mouth to the back of the throat, but the other 99 percent of your body is begging for you to stop poisoning it. The average American consumed 39 pounds of high-fructose corn syrup in 1980 and 62.6 pounds in 2001. It is being considered as one of the major contributors to obesity in America. Hmmmmm, good.

The third ingredient I want to mention is aspartame and other artificial sweeteners such as sucralose. Aspartame affects the brain and makes you crave carbohydrates. Most soda beverages that are called "diet" contain these ingredients. There have been numerous reports on the dangers of these sweeteners, but somehow they have been kept in thousands of products, and people are getting fatter and fatter eating these so-called "diet" products.

Again, "You are what you don't eat" is as powerful as "You are what you eat." By simply getting rid of these ingredients, you will notice that many of the dangerous weight-causing foods that you eat will be eliminated from your diet, and you will begin to look for better choices. It is when you make this transformation that you begin to push out the old toxins from your system and your body starts to crave better foods.

Another form of detoxification is adding fiber to your diet. As a nation, we do not eat enough fiber, because we are not eating enough live foods. Fiber will help clean the digestive system. The fiber helps detoxify the colon, which many will agree is the starting place of most disease. So many people are dehydrated and constipated. This is such a fatal combination for bad health. I myself increased my fiber intake not only with fruits and vegetables, but also with psyllium husks and oats. I even went as far as getting a colon hydrotherapy. At the time I received it, I lost about two pounds from the process. I had already been eating properly for about eight months, so the hydrotherapist even told me I was very clean inside. Some people, though, have so much backed-up fecal matter that they are artificially up to thirty pounds overweight. John Wayne and Elvis Presley both were reported to have many pounds of undigested fecal matter in their systems when they died. I had read that John Wayne had up to forty pounds of undigested fecal matter in his system. This certainly is not healthy, and we know more about it today perhaps than we did back then. Constipation is a huge deal, and everything you can do to prevent it will lead towards greater health. It certainly has for me.

Another step in the detox process is to add more berries to your diet. Berries have antioxidants, which fight free radicals in your system that cause aging. They also are loaded with nutrients that I can't even pronounce. The deep colors of berries and their great taste are evidence of their power to give your body some of the nutrients it needs to fight off disease. Berries should be a number one staple in everyone's diet. In the winter, you can get frozen organic berries and add them to your smoothies to make them cold. The freezing process may have an effect on the overall level of nutrient availability in food, so it is always best to have raw and unfrozen berries, but I find the convenience of the frozen berries worth it for myself.

The next phase I focused on was the liver and bacteria in my system. I knew that even though I had a hydrotherapy, that my digestive system may have had organisms living there that shouldn't be there, and I knew my liver had taken a beating from alcohol. I started to drink herbal teas that contained milk thistle and dandelion root, which I had researched were good liver detoxifiers. I also began to eat spices such as turmeric more often. Turmeric is a fantastic spice which is getting a lot of attention in the media. Anytime a real food that grows and has been used by ancient civilizations for centuries starts to get a lot of attention in the West, I take notice. It's unfortunate that we are so behind in these areas, but the way I see it is that I need to take notice of what is going on in this arena and seek out the information proactively, so I can make informed, intelligent choices as to how I want to consume them. I start out with a little, and if I feel better as a result, I add a little more.

Lemon water is also a gentle liver cleanse, as are powerful foods such as garlic, onions, and ginger. Again, all of these foods grow in nature and survive the roughest of conditions. Besides the fiber in my digestive system, I also began to take probiotics. Your system needs to balance out the good bacteria and bad bacteria in your digestive tract. I noticed a great difference in my energy levels when I started to take probiotics. I believe my system began to function better and absorb foods better when it became more in balance. I also began to take black walnut hull, which comes from the inside of a walnut shell and is available as a supplement. It is used to flush out stubborn bacteria and parasites that hang around the digestive tract.

Another great addition to my diet was supplemental enzymes. I felt that my system had suffered a toll over the past few years from all that meat and processed foods, and, quite frankly, my system needed some help digesting. Enzymes are reported to be supportive in so many of our essential life functions, but I took them as a digestive aid and as an anti-inflammatory. I believe that inflammation is one of the causes of many of our health problems, and the more I can do to eliminate inflammation, the better my body is going to be able to stay healthy. My cardiovascular system suffered a toll over the years. I was a smoker for a few years as a teenager and then for a few months in my twenties when I was back on alcohol. I also would get bronchitis and sinus infections all the time, and I suspected I had tissue damage deep in my lungs. Exercising is certainly therapeutic for cardiovascular detoxification and was certainly a main step that I used. The deeper we breathe and the more oxygen we get in our lungs, the better our lungs are going to function. Eating greens and cucumbers also helps detoxify the lungs. Moving on to the kidneys, I had always heard that drinking water was one of the best ways to detoxify the kidneys. Ginger is also helpful, as are cranberries. Once a year, I will try to do more detoxing than usual for a few weeks straight. I will eat less and take in a lot of the foods mentioned earlier. A lot has been said about fasting and minimizing the consumption of food as a way to increase life span. One of the reasons for this is probably that we take in fewer toxins if we eat less. We also generate more human growth hormones when we eat less, and certain genes are affected positively when we eat less. The amount of oxidative stress is reduced by our not taking in as many free radicals, and this in itself causes a reduction of inflammation. Inflammation is just another cause of pain as far as I'm concerned, and it affects our health in many ways. As an athlete, I want to do everything I can to keep inflammation down so that I can perform at peak levels. It therefore is important for me to take antioxidant-rich foods and supplements.

Genes!

I used to always give in to the gene theory, and it affected the way I thought. I know many people feel that their genes determine their destiny, but in most cases it is food that triggers your genes' behavior. I believe in the theory that it is not family history that affects your health, but your family eating habits. Most generations follow the foods that their families have eaten. I have chosen to research what the most awesome foods in the world are and to get as much of those foods as possible. One of the tests that I did to find clues to improving my health was to get a gene profile. You can have a swab test done to look at your gene variations and to get insight into potential areas which you could be affected by if you eat the wrong foods. The study of nutritional genomics has come a long way, and can be a great addition to your arsenal of knowledge. Nutrition is just one factor, however, in the ways your genes are affected. All of your lifestyle choices—the environments you put yourself into, the ways you think and handle stress, and how much exercise you do—all play a role. There is already proof of certain nutrients that have an effect on genes. Lycopene, which is found in tomato products, has been found to slow down a gene responsible for prostate cancer. Curcumin suppresses genes associated with inflammation. Curcumin is found in turmeric, which has been recently studied as a possible cancer inhibitor. Omega-3 fatty acids have long been known to inhibit inflammation-causing genes. Cruciferous vegetables have been shown to help with genes involved in the detoxification process. So if your genes are weak in the detoxification area, then cruciferous vegetables may help. Others, as we know, have great detoxification genes and can drink alcohol and smoke until they are ninety. This is rare, because even though one set of genes perform better, there could be others that don't—so one way or the other, a bad diet will catch up with you. We all know this, don't we? None of this is new information. In fact, what if it was truly proven beyond a shadow of a doubt and made public that you can live to 150 years old by eating fruits, vegetables, and superfoods daily? Would people do it? I think that subconsciously, most people know what the answer to great health is, but it is their addictive behaviors and their inability to control them and feel happiness without them that prevents the change. That's why I believe a superfood awakening is the path towards making a lifestyle change. Once you resign yourself to the notion that you are what you eat and you start to view it as a medicine of some sort, then you truly open the door to change which can be sustained.

Organic foods and superfoods bring along with them a high-frequency vibration that only our bodies understand. I believe this frequency can be seen, as I mentioned earlier, with Kirlian photography. Below is a picture of an organic raw cacao bean. If the picture doesn't at least make you wonder, what in the world is that energy field around the food? How did it get there? What significance does it have when we swallow that cacao bean?

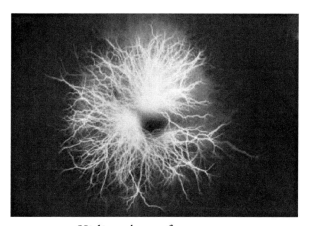

Kirlian photo of raw cacao

I believe it has tremendous significance, as does eating organic food versus nonorganic food. Organic food is grown with love. The soils are kept rich with minerals, and therefore the plant grows in a healthy environment. In order for produce to be certified as organic, the farmer must not use pesticides, fungicides, herbicides, or any other pollutants. The crop yield is usually lower, and therefore the cost of organic food is higher. However, you may not pay as much of a monetary price for nonorganic food, but eventually you will pay later as your body has to deal with the excess toxins. Organic food, by some reports, can have up to 300 percent more nutrients than nonorganic food.

Chapter 8 - The light bulb starts to flicker

One of the goals for this book is to spark a superfood awakening in you. I want to turn on that light bulb inside of you. I want to wake up that inner component that will give you the strength and inspiration you need to see the possibilities that are right in front of us. Some people call it an "aha" moment, some call it an epiphany, and some call it a good kick in the butt. Call it what you want, but in the end you will get a completely different outlook on what is most important in life. And to me, that's an energetic, passionately inspired *you*. We talked a little about cleansing and how important it is as one of the first steps in cleaning house. I like to look at it as pulling the plug on the bathtub. Once the internal environment is cleaned a little, we have something to work with us instead of against us. That's what I did. I started with drinking higher-pH water. I eliminated alcohol, minimized coffee intake, and got rid of fast food, processed foods, dairy products, and meats. I began to eat more vegetables and fruits. I became acquainted with fruits that I didn't even know were fruits, such as avocados. I had never eaten a raw avocado. Now I eat about three or four a week. Avocadoes are great sprinkled with sea salt and dulse and a little organic lemon juice. They have protein and good plant-based fats high in essential fatty acids that we need.

I personally believe that as humans on planet earth, we are capable at this point of living to 125 years old and beyond. It is a shame that many people will not reach this age because the odds are stacked against most people. Where I want to take the rest of this book is to give all the tools I think can be used to achieve optimal health. I am going to list all of the foods I believe will help stack the odds in your favor, as well as all the lifestyle changes. Although I am not listing them in any particular order, I do believe that the concepts listed earlier are going to give you the biggest bang for your buck, so to speak, in helping you achieve longevity. I can tell you that they are the steps that I am following and that are working for me. I am hoping that one of the steps listed will give you your own superfood awakening. Maybe it's a superfood that you really connect with or a lifestyle change that you connect with so deeply that you start to research it more deeply. You then in your research discover other concepts that you were unaware of, and this snowball effect starts to get you angry that you were not aware of these ideas previously. You then become more educated and continue to seek out new information and share it with others that you know and care about. You can take health to any level that you want. For some, this may mean taking the simplest path in order to get the biggest effect. For those, I recommend doing four things and eliminating four things (see below). For the rest, I recommend taking this entire book and doing all that you can do, all that you are willing to do, and all that you are able to do.

Tips for the individual who wants it to be as easy as possible

Top four things to add or increase

1 – Add more fruits, superfoods, and vegetables, and have them every day (organic if possible, most days of the week)
2 – Eat whole grains (quinoa, spelt, amaranth, wheat, millet, steel-cut oats, brown rice (organic if possible most days of the week)
3 – Eat essential fats most meals (avocados, olive oil, nuts, and seeds) (organic if possible most days of the week)
4 – Exercise and drink half your weight in ounces per day or more

(If you do not get the calories you need from the above four steps, you can add other sources of protein of your choice, such as fish and poultry and legumes. All the essential amino acids, which are the building blocks of proteins, are available in fruits, vegetables, and grains; however, it is a reality that many people do not desire to get all their calories from fruits, vegetables, superfoods, and grains. You also have to make sure you are getting vitamin B_{12}, iron, calcium, zinc, and protein in adequate amounts as a vegetarian or raw foodist. A two-thousand-calorie or more diet seems to be adequate for most people. Exercise requires you to add enough calories to replace what you are burning off in that exercise session. There are resources available online related to calories burned for different types of exercises based on your body weight. I have also used www.nutritiondata.com as a great source for nutrient information. For instance, sesame seeds and broccoli are both good sources of calcium, ounce for ounce, compared to milk.)

Top four things to not do or to drastically reduce (I did)

1 – Eliminate partially hydrogenated oils (trans fats) (check the labels)
2 – Eliminate high-fructose corn syrup, aspartame, and other processed sugars
3 – Eliminate processed salts, preservatives, and dyes
4 – Eliminate nicotine and reduce caffeine and alcohol

Chapter 8 – Will Power's
Lifestyle Choices

Tips for living to 125 years old and beyond for those who want to achieve the highest level of health. (Tips I follow)

Stay alkaline

Have you ever heard of the expression "Money is energy" or "Everything is energy"? Energy comes from many places, such as emotional uplift, adrenaline, and biological processes at the cellular level, but at the core it is the state of someone's acid-alkaline balance. There are some individuals who seem to be genetically alkaline. You know, those people that are endless chatterboxes, who seem to be able to drink twelve martinis and eat large portions of rich, fatty foods, and can still survive on five hours' sleep. There are also even more people who are genetically acidic and seem to always be carrying around a bottle of Tums. Everything seems to bother their stomachs, especially citrus drinks made with high-fructose corn syrup, alcohol, coffee, and large meals with red meat (you know, the twenty-eight-ounce porterhouse). The good news for someone who tends to be more acidic is that you can help the body bring up your pH level with the proper diet. The bad news for high-alkaline individuals is that, although they may be peak performers for many years and enjoy extremely high energy, they also tend to be very prone to heart attacks at young ages, since they tend to eat a very acidic diet that overloads the blood vessels around the heart.

The acid-alkaline balance is also known as the body's pH level. Your blood is constantly trying to maintain a pH of about 7.4. Do you remember chemistry class when you stuck that piece of litmus paper in the different liquids? A pH of 7.0 is neutral. A pH above 7.0 is alkaline, and a pH below 7.0 is acidic. Coffee, alcohol, colas, red meat, sugar, many sweetened fruit juices and canned fruits, beans, dairy products, most grains and nuts are largely on the acidic side. Vegetables, fish, healthy oils, and raw fruits are more alkaline-forming. Most people think that lemons are acidic. Although the lemon itself has a low pH, when it is swallowed, digested, and assimilated, it is alkaline-forming in the body.

How important is the concept of pH? If blood pH moves below 6.8 or above 7.8, cells stop functioning and the body dies. I would say it is extremely important. Unfortunately, the Standard American Diet (SAD) is very acidic, and foods are not the only things that cause us to live in a state of acidosis. Stress, extreme exercise, environmental toxins, and anything that deprives the cells of oxygen—such as improper breathing or poorly ventilated buildings—will make us more acidic.

Our bodies are amazing, and when we become acidic, there are mechanisms which work to keep us alkaline. Minerals such as sodium, calcium, magnesium, and potassium—which are some of the most alkaline substances on the planet—are robbed from other areas of our bodies, such as organs and bones. This state of acidosis has been proven to be a leading cause of arthritis, osteoporosis, bronchitis, nasal infections, and many other illnesses. Research has even shown that cancer cannot survive in an alkaline environment. I personally suffered from bronchitis and nasal infections, as well as arthritic conditions, for many years. I believe there were two reasons for this:

1. An overly acidic diet
2. Participating in extreme sports such as marathons, triathlons, track-and-field, and cross-country racing without the knowledge of how to stay alkaline

Many people are unaware of the acid-forming oxidative effects that extreme exercise has on their bodies. Cyclists are seen with runny noses while riding their bikes. The oxidative effects of lactic acid buildup, combined with having an acidic body, forces the body to react and remove the toxic buildup. It can be a tendency for people who exercise to feel invincible and feel that they can eat anything they want because of their cardiovascular or muscular fitness. I would say the opposite is true; we can never escape the truth that you are what you eat. An athlete, in particular, needs to take on even more measures than most to continually make the body alkaline with vegetable juices, high-alkaline water, and minerals. Many health practitioners believe in taking small amounts of sodium bicarbonate (baking soda) when one feels the onset of stuffiness or a cold to help increase the body's alkaline state. Herbal teas, lemon and water, and increasing sea salt and calcium intake will also help. Practicing deep breathing can also help in many ways. Many people do not breathe deeply enough or exercise and therefore are not using their entire lung capacity. Toxins can build up in the lower portions of the lungs over time, which can lead to lung infections and coughing. When oxygen enters the full lung, one can feel the energy almost immediately. Coincidently, oxygen is extremely alkaline. I truly believe that keeping the body alkaline is one of the most important aspects of health, wellness, and longevity.

Eat green

Eating green is in line with staying alkaline, because greens are some of the most alkaline foods on the planet because they are rich in minerals. Green foods contain chlorophyll, enzymes, minerals, vitamins, water, phytonutrients, and many yet-to-be-discovered wonders which keep our bodies functioning. Awesome green foods include kale, spinach, broccoli, lettuce, cucumber, celery, kelp, endive, and bok choy. There is nothing more amazing for your body than green foods made by the sun. The life force energy and high mineralization of these foods make them a number one priority for longevity.

Eat organic

Organic foods contain many nutrients and are certified to contain no harmful pesticides or fungicides. When you eat organic foods, you are getting food that is richer in minerals, has more energy inherent in the food, and contains more nutrients than foods which are not organic. If you are a meat eater and buy organic meats, then you are getting food from animals that have been fed organic grasses and foods and have not been treated with hormones or antibiotics which ultimately get passed on to you. However, keep in mind that if there is anything to say about the nutritional value of meat, it is because of the grasses and plants that the animals are eating. I sometimes say to myself, *Why process the plants through the animal and eat the animal? Why not go straight to the source and get it before it has been processed through the animal?* I remember the first time I really "got it" in regards to organic foods and their enormous benefits. I was standing in a supermarket which sold primarily organic food products called Whole Foods Market. I had just finished a long run and was just looking for something healthy to eat. I walked through the produce section and was in awe at the amazing beauty of the fruits and vegetables as the misty filtered water sprayed them as if in slow motion. The purple, green, and red kale, in particular, were as alive as if they had not yet been picked. In fact, green, leafy vegetables are indeed breathing, living organic substances. They are packed with chlorophyll, which is nearly identical to the hemoglobin in human blood. It is for this reason that green, leafy vegetables are perhaps the greatest single food on the face of the earth.

Introducing organic foods into your diet just may be the answer you are looking for that no one will tell you about. When I say no one, I mean the people you are currently seeking out for advice on your health. Unless you are going to a wellness professional that has dedicated his or her life to the prevention of sickness and the healing of mankind, the chances of your getting an empathetic response in regards to your own extreme health are diminished.

Organic foods are certified to be free of pesticides, herbicides, and fungicides. They are grown with love and respect, verse greed and disrespect. Organic foods in essence are as close to your natural makeup as you can get. They are richer in nutrients and minerals. Vegetables are richer in chlorophyll and enzymes. Fruits are richer in antioxidants and flavonoids. Organic grains are not polluted with chemicals sprayed on them just so they don't fall down from having so many pesticides sprayed on them. Do you think that by ingesting some of this clean, pure food your chances of living longer are greater? I say yes, and I back it up with my own experiences of feeling vibrant health ever since I introduced organic foods into my diet. Not only have all my health-related stats come into normal areas, but I went from not being able to walk up a flight of stairs to training for an Ironman triathlon. So many people take advantage of their health, not realizing that they are one Twinkie away from toxicity.

By introducing organic foods into your diet, you will help your body eliminate the toxins found in nonorganic foods. These toxins are really hard on the immune system—including your lymphatic system—your blood, your liver, your gall bladder, and your entire cardiovascular system. If you are not cleansing, you are at further risk of toxic buildup in the form of bloated fat cells, which is where your body will tend to safely store toxic overload.

Drink high-pH water

In Tip #1, we talked about staying alkaline. If we are to stay alkaline, then the nutrient we need more of than any other needs to be alkaline (have a high pH). Our bodies are made up of primarily water. Water is critical to all life functions. Most people take it for granted and do not drink enough. Sometimes, it's because of their busy lifestyle; yet, what is the priority? I actually hear people say, "I drink coffee all day, so I don't need water." Caffeine can actually cause dehydration and increase water needs. Decaffeinated coffee is so chemically processed that it may be worse for you than regular coffee is. We should drink approximately half our weight in ounces per day. However, if you are sedentary (not active and sitting at a desk all day) and you find yourself needing to go take a potty break too often, then consume less water, because too much water can leach your body of minerals in which it is already deficient. A high-pH water such as Fiji (about 7.5 pH), Evamore (9.0 pH), and Iceland Spring about (8.25 pH) will help keep you hydrated and alkaline, which may ultimately give you more energy. Spring water is probably the best source of water, but unless you bottle it yourself at the source, you will have to drink it from plastic-leaching water bottles. Reverse osmosis–filtered water has been reported to be better for you than plain, nonfiltered tap water, because most of the chemicals are filtered out. Distilled water is pure H_2O and is a great source of water, but it is also demineralized, so you would want to replace those minerals and perhaps ionize the water to give it its life force energy back. Dehydration is a major cause of many issues that people deal with, such as constipation, poor skin, lack of energy, and fevers.

Explore enzyme supplements

As an athlete, I know the power of taking enzyme supplements as a great anti-inflammatory, as a digestive aid, and as a cleansing aid. Enzymes have so many great advantages that everyone should consider taking them as a longevity aid. Neither vitamins, minerals, nor hormones can do any work without enzymes. We are born with a certain potential for creating enzymes. We can also consume enzymes through raw, living foods; however, most people live on cooked foods. Enzymes are destroyed at above 118 degrees Fahrenheit. Enzyme deficiencies are believed by some experts to be a paramount cause of premature aging and early death. Our digestive systems are constantly robbing our supplies of enzymes to digest cooked foods, leaving the rest of our organs and metabolic processes starving for enzymes. Find a great source of enzymes such as Beauty Enzymes (at http://sunfood.com/Catalog/Default.aspx). These enzymes are magnificent and some of the best on the planet.

An understanding of the importance of enzymes might just be one of the key elements missing in one's awareness of optimal health. When I first heard about enzymes, I had no idea what they were. I had a clue that they had something to do with digestion, but I felt there was more to this miracle biological element. In fact, the more I have learned about enzymes, the more I am convinced that they are probably one of the most important elements in a lifestyle which lends itself to super-nutrition.

When we put food or liquids into our mouths, the enzymatic process begins to break down foods. This process continues in the stomach and the small intestine and is critical to breaking down foods so that the nutrients in the food can be broken down and absorbed. These nutrients include fats, proteins, carbohydrates, vitamins, and minerals. If our bodies are not able to absorb the nutrients, we feel weak, tired, and unfulfilled. Why wouldn't our bodies be able to absorb the nutrients?

There are several reasons:

1. The food we are eating does not contain the nutrients, either because the food was overcooked and the nutrients were partially destroyed or because the food was grown in nutrient-deficient soil.
2. Our bodies lack the necessary enzymes because the biological processes that produce the enzymes have been compromised and overloaded with toxins.

Every time we put food or liquids into our mouth, we are indeed making a choice as to how we want to live our life. Foods that are deficient in enzymes force the body to overwork itself to produce what is needed to break down the foods. Have you ever wondered why people take naps after they eat? The body is overworking to digest the food which has been consumed. Most people will not feel exhausted after eating an organic salad and fruit which are rich in enzymes.

Why else are enzymes so important? Just as important as their role in digestion, enzymes are the key that transport nutrients into our cells. They transport the nutrients throughout our body and bring them to where they are needed. And what might possibly be the most important thing about enzymes is that when enzymes do not have anything else to do in the digestive tract, they become like soldiers moving around the body, working on inflammation. This can be a huge concept in our understanding of health and nutrition, especially for very active athletes, who frequently are inflamed after workouts. I personally take enzyme supplements such as bromelain and papain once or twice a day or after a hard race or workout. Papayas are high in the enzyme papain, and pineapples are high in the enzyme bromelain. These enzymes can also be purchased in supplemental form. It is important to get high-quality supplements if you want to take enzymes in supplemental form, and they should be taken with food if you eat a lot of cooked foods (which most people do). You can also take them on an empty stomach, and they have a cleansing effect on the body, as they will perform like little Pacmen that go around the body repairing tissue and reducing inflammation.

If you really want to get the most benefit from enzymes and their amazing effects on the human body, get them from fresh squeezed vegetable and fruit juices. You can go to your whole food grocers, who can juice them for you on the spot using cucumbers, carrots, celery, beets, kale, parsley, etc. You will not only get the squeezed-out enzymes, but you will also be getting the vitamins, minerals, and chlorophyll which will help keep your body in an alkaline state and as vibrant as ever.

Consume more fiber

Everyone tells you to eat more fiber. Why? There are many benefits to fiber, and I believe the most important is its ability to keep the digestive engine clean. If your digestive tract is clogged with undigested food, it is more difficult to absorb nutrients. Many autopsies have revealed twenty pounds or more of undigested fecal matter in people that have died. This even made news with famous people such as

John Wayne and Elvis Presley, as was mentioned previously. There is a reason the gut starts to push out as we age. Most people are eating large quantities of unhealthy nonorganic red meats, not enough fiber from fruits and vegetables, processed hydrogenated foods, and high-glycemic processed sugars, and the intestines build up a protective barrier over time to block the unhealthy bits of chemicals, hormones, antibiotics, and pesticides that these foods contain. A great way to get fiber besides fruits and vegetables is from hemp seeds, flaxseeds, raw steel-cut oats, and psyllium husks. I add these to my smoothies in the morning to get an extra ten grams a day. Men need approximately thirty-eight grams a day, and women need about twenty-five grams.

Consume high-quality omega-3 oils

This is certainly one of my top ten longevity tips. Omega-3's are great for the heart, great for your joints through their anti-inflammatory properties, and have special properties to help our brains function. Most people associate omega-3's with fish. Be careful, because there is a reason why plastic bag use has made the news. Plastic bags are polluting our oceans, and they are not what they used to be ten thousand years ago. Also, a lot of the fish is farm-raised in big tanks unless it is labeled wild-caught. Not all fish oils are the same, either. You have to know the source of the fish that the oil comes from. Anchovies and sardines tend to have lower mercury levels and could be better than larger fish. Better yet, you can get your omega-3's where I get them, which is from organic cold-pressed olive oil, hemp seed oil and hemp seeds, flaxseed oil and flaxseeds, raw organic olives, avocados and nuts, krill oil, and marine phytoplankton.

Occasionally, I will have wild-caught Norwegian salmon oil.

Explore probiotics

Probiotics are starting to become well known. If you have ever taken antibiotics, then some of your good bacteria, or probiotics, have been destroyed. Probiotics help kill off unwanted bacteria and keep your digestive system healthier. The digestive system is the heart of your core. Everything you are evolves around it, because you are what you eat. Every cell in your body is made up of what you put in your mouth—garbage in, garbage out, so to speak. Probiotics can be taken in supplemental form as an aid in keeping the digestive system healthy. There are also certain foods such as goji berries that have good bacteria in them inherently. Without a healthy digestive system, it doesn't matter how much you can bench press or if you can run a five-minute mile. Your body will feel the effects of it over a few years as your new cells are made up of unhealthy substances passing through your digestive tract that are not stopped and end up in your bloodstream and lymphatic system.

Reduce stress

Stress is certainly a killer. You can put on weight from binge eating as a result of stress. Stress takes on many forms that most people are not aware of. Extreme exercise creates oxidative stress, pollution creates environmental stress, and loud noises create primitive responses of stress which make you "jump" and temporarily stress your adrenals and create cortisol. Your body is affected at a cellular level when you are stressed. There is a reason your hair stands up on your arms when you are scared. Your brain, nervous system, thoughts, and emotions are all connected to your cells. The ability to control stress has been proven to help prevent aging. Easier said than done is what I say. We all have had the tailgater driver come up behind us because we weren't going fast enough for him. Deep breathing is a great stress reliever and the easiest and cheapest to do yourself. Take ten deep breaths, preferably outdoors, a couple of times a day. You can also do it at night while lying in bed before sleep. This is a cheap form of meditation that works for me. Yoga is also a great way, as are all forms of light exercise. Extreme exercise does add stress to the body in certain ways. If you are an athlete, you have to take extra measures, such as increasing antioxidant intake, staying alkaline, staying hydrated, keeping limber and flexible, taking care of your joints with natural anti-inflammatories, and taking adequate recovery periods. The older we get, the more important this is, because we do not recover from stress as well as when we were teenagers or in our twenties and thirties.

Make two very important decisions correctly

The way we live our life has a lot to do with wellness and longevity. Probably the two most important decisions you will ever make is who you marry or partner with and what you do as your vocation (job or business) or passion. Your lifestyle is affected by the people you spend the most time with, as are your stress levels and habits. The divorce rate is over 60 percent, and people are constantly changing jobs as they try to find their passion. All these life events contribute to stress on the body. Make it a priority to marry yourself first. Find out who you are and love yourself; then you will be able to align yourself with the right person and the passion that drives you every day for a healthier and fruitful life.

Eat superfoods

What is a superfood? I often get this question when I mention that my diet consists primarily of organic foods and in particular organic superfoods. Superfoods are foods which are extremely nutrient dense and give you the biggest bang for your buck compared to other foods. They contain amazing medicinal-like properties in that they have been used in different cultures for thousands of years for healing, for endurance, for vibrant health, and for their so-called antiaging and longevity characteristics. They usually are high in antioxidants and minerals as well as being enzyme rich. There are different levels of superfoods. In fact, some superfoods are very well known, and most people do not realize they are eating what has been "labeled" as a superfood. By labeled, I mean that they are sometimes marketed as superfoods because there tends to be some evidence that the foods are a healthier alternative to most foods. Perhaps this is true, but in fact, a true superfood will be at its healthiest state when it is in its raw, uncooked form. Foods often marketed as superfoods include foods such as garlic, broccoli, kale, tomatoes, papaya, spinach, parsley, oats, turkey, eggs, walnuts, pumpkin, almonds, figs, chili peppers, cayenne pepper, pomegranate, blueberries, raspberries, and wild salmon. Some of these are in fact extremely healthy foods, and in some cases like garlic, they are as close to being superfoods as they can be. Many of us have heard of these foods and have eaten them time and time again. It is certainly better to get the organic or wild variety of these foods, in that they are even more "super" without the added chemicals and preservatives.

Some other superfoods are not as well known. These are the foods which can get you to the next level of extreme health. I have spent the last couple of years researching some of these superfoods, which I consider to be some of the best foods in the world and have used in my daily diet with tremendous success. These superfoods which I am about to talk about are absolutely amazing and have helped cultures for thousands of years avoid famine and disease. Kings and queens would go to war to get more of these superfoods. For instance, it has been said that Alexander the Great was persuaded by Aristotle to invade Egypt for the aloe vera plant so he could use it on his injured soldiers. Back then, we didn't have clinical studies to tell us what was good and bad for us. They used foods to treat people, and they either worked or didn't work. This process over thousands of years brought notice of these greatest of superfoods and herbs to the leaders of great countries.

The following are some of the greatest superfoods I have learned about over the last several years, which are available on the Internet as well as at local health food stores.

Hemp seeds and hemp protein – These contain omega-3 and omega-6 essential fatty acids in an ideal proportion. They are a complete protein, meaning they contain all the essential amino acids and an abundance of trace minerals which we are deficient in as a society.

Bee pollen – Bee pollen has been used since way back in the ancient Chinese and Egyptian civilizations and has an incredible array of vitamins, minerals, amino acids, enzymes, and coenzymes. It is especially rich in B vitamins and antioxidants, including lycopene, selenium, beta-carotene, vitamin C, vitamin E, and several flavonoids. It is composed of 55 percent carbohydrates, 35 percent protein, 3 percent vitamins and minerals, 2 percent fatty acids, and 5 percent other substances. Overall, it's one of the most nutritionally complete natural substances found on earth.

Maca powder – This is a natural adaptogen that helps the body combat stress. It has endurance- and stamina-enhancing properties and is a well-known aphrodisiac in that it helps improve sexual function in men and women

Spirulina – This is a food which fed Mexico City for thousands of years. It is the highest source of protein on the planet (62 percent protein). It is great mixed with just plain spring water or juice.

Blue-green algae – This is another great ocean superfood rich in amino acids (also a complete plant-based protein), enzymes, antioxidants, and minerals. Blue-green algae is also a rich source of calcium, iron, and vitamin B_{12}.

Chlorella – Chlorella is also a great open-water food. It is a natural detoxifier of heavy metals and pesticides. It is good for the digestive system, is high in protein and magnesium, and is a great cleansing food. It can be purchased in powder or capsule form.

Marine phytoplankton – Some three and a half billion years ago, the appearance of tiny organisms with the ability to convert sunlight, oxygen, water, and minerals into protein, carbohydrates, vitamins, and amino acids began to appear. These tiny organisms are called phytoplankton, the single-cell plants that are the basis of all other life forms on planet earth. Phytoplankton are responsible for making up to 90 percent of Earth's oxygen. Phytoplankton are the food utilized by the world's largest and longest-living animals and fish. Blue whales, bowhead whales, and many other types of whales all eat plankton. These species live to between 80 and 150 years old and maintain great strength throughout their lives.

Sprouts – Sprouts are one of the most nutritionally dense live foods on the planet. This made a lot of sense to me when I first learned about sprouts. When a seed or bean sprout is at its most active enzymatic state, it is richest in minerals, proteins, and vitamins. They are also rich in chlorophyll. Most people have heard of store-bought alfalfa or bean sprouts that are used on salads; however, it is simple to grow sprouts using a simple hemp seed bag or grower in your home.

Wheatgrass and barley grass – Grasses are also some of the most nutrient-dense, mineral-rich, enzyme-active foods on the planet. They are as close to the soil as you can get. Horses thrive on grasses, as do organic cattle, for a reason. You can grow your own in trays, you can get wheatgrass shots at a whole foods market, or you can get the powdered form and add them to smoothies.

Dulse and kelp– These are nutritious seaweed vegetables packed with minerals, vitamins, and antioxidants.

Goji berries – Goji berries are another complete protein source. They are high in antioxidants, iron, and vitamin C, and they contain twenty-one trace minerals and many other nutrients. They are small, light, and portable. I usually eat just one handful of goji berries before a cross-country flight and do not have to eat anything the entire flight.

Cacao beans – Cacao beans are the actual raw chocolate bean, which most people have never eaten. Most are familiar with the processed version of cacao called cocoa or chocolate, which is mostly sugar and dairy mixed together with the cacao bean. Cacao is one of the highest antioxidants on the ORAC scale known to date. (The ORAC scale measures the level of antioxidant power in foods)

Organic MSM – MSM (Methylsulfonylmethane) supplies sulfur to the body, which allows it to heal itself. It produces muscle relaxation and reduces swelling.

Avocados – The avocado is a rich fruit high in the good fats called monounsaturated fats. They are also high in potassium, calcium, vitamins C and K, copper, folic acid, and fiber. Avocados—along with olive oil, nuts, and seeds—are my first choice for the 20 percent of your calories that should come from healthy fats.

Coconut and coconut oil – Coconut is highly nutritious and rich in fiber, vitamins, and minerals. It is high in a plant-based saturated fat and contains medium-chain triglycerides, which provide an immediate source of energy. We need saturated fats in small amounts for our skin, but it needs to come from a plant-based source, and coconut oil is one of the best food sources to get them from.

Acai berries – The acai berry is a berry from the Amazon rain forest; the major benefits of the acai berry are thought to include its heart health benefits. The acai berry is known to be a rich source of compounds called anthocyanins. These anthocyanins are the same compounds thought to give red wine its health benefits, yet the acai berry has none of the health risks associated with alcohol. The acai berry is also a rich source of protein and dietary fiber, in addition to having high levels of both omega-6 and omega-9 fatty acids.

Mangosteen – There have been numerous studies related to the health benefits of this exotic fruit. I like it for its anti-inflammatory properties, but it has also been said to be anticarcinogenic, antifungal, and a powerful antioxidant.

Royal jelly – This is a food given to the queen bee by worker bees and is filled with vitamins, minerals, proteins, and fatty acids.

Flaxseeds – A great food to add to smoothies, this seed is rich in fatty acids, manganese, magnesium, and fiber.

Green tea – Rich in antioxidants and a staple in Japanese culture, green tea is a staple treat in my diet. The green matcha variety which I use is used in the sacred Japanese tea ceremony called Chado.

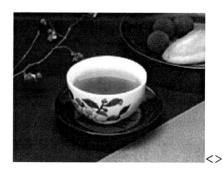

Cordyceps – Cordyceps is a medicinal mushroom known for its immune system–enhancing properties and its ability to significantly increase maximal oxygen uptake and the anaerobic threshold, which may lead to improved exercise capacity and resistance to fatigue.

Most of these superfoods can be obtained in powdered form and added to your favorite super-smoothie in the morning. You will get just about every vitamin, mineral, amino acid, good fat (omega-3, -6, and -9), and hundreds of other phytonutrients and glyconutrients by eating these foods. Every longevity and antiaging diet should not be without these superfoods. Athletes, in particular, whose bodies are hungry for antioxidants, anti-inflammatories, and minerals, should incorporate these foods into their diet.

You are what you don't eat

In the first ten tips, we talked about a lot of things we should do. With most people, there is a lot they could do by just stopping what they are doing. No one wants to be told what to do. For whatever reason, we are all rebels within. Like kids, you tell us what to do and we do the opposite. Sometimes, however, we hear something that we do not take personally. We actually connect with it and a voice goes off that says, "I didn't know that. If I knew that, I would have never eaten that or did that or bought that." Here are a few tips that by themselves will change your health for the better, if you indeed have the passion to change your health. Go through your closets and refrigerator and look for anything with the following ingredients (we will discuss them in more detail later): high-fructose corn syrup, hydrogenated oils (of any kind), aspartame, MSG (monosodium glutamate), natural flavoring and dyes, spices (both of these labeling techniques are very generic ways for the food companies to legally put preservatives in food), bleached flours, enriched flours, any other word you just don't understand that the food doctors have added to make you say, "Mmmmm, tastes good, so who cares if it's bad for me." Also look for carbonated beverages, colas, caffeinated beverages, microwaved food, fast food, alcoholic beverages, and the hardest of all, over time—all nonorganic foods. I know you are not going to be able to do this all at once. Over time, though, if you did, you would move towards great health. So realize that it is a choice. You don't have to do it 100 percent. I understand that dramatic changes throw people out of balance and they need to start out with one meal a week being healthy then move to one meal a day. It took me about three months to implement all of the above. I still eat nonorganic at times when I cheat, but I don't feel guilty because it's just 5 percent of the time. The hardest was coffee, but I replaced it with fifteen different kinds of teas (yes, I have an addictive personality) that I could explore and experiment with—such as ginseng tea, green tea, yerba maté, dandelion root, milk thistle, and chamomile. Introduce one great food a week, and get rid of one bad food a week. You don't have to do this if it will stress you out. If that is the case, you are better off living the way you are in a way that suits you. However, if you feel something can be changed, then at a minimum, as you eat the good stuff it will "crowd out" the bad stuff. You will naturally reduce cravings as you increase the nutrient-dense foods. There are a lot of diets out there that stress certain percentages of each food group. Perhaps the best percentage is when you eat good food most of the time; then when the bad stuff works its way in, it is such a small percentage that it will not bring on guilt and shame. Over time, you will see the results and you will be pulled naturally to the better lifestyle.

Research colonics

Visit a naturopathic professional and ask about the benefits of a colonic. It's what I call "unclogging the drain." So many people have all these symptoms of acid reflux, lethargy, cramps, constipation, weird pains which they can't describe, lack of energy—symptoms which they explain to their doctor which results in all these tests being done with no solution. My studies have indicated that over 90 percent of diseases start in the intestines and colon. That is where your "second heart" is, so to speak. Everything you eat is passing through there (and a lot of it isn't). In fact, some of it stays there for a very long time, and some of it even leaches into other parts of your body. A colonic is a first step towards lightening the load and getting rid of residue, toxins, and hardened fecal matter that have built up inside you. Educate yourself about the process and its benefits. Commit to getting a colonic yearly or at a frequency recommended by your naturopathic professional.

Avoid or reduce meats

There are certainly many meat eaters among us who may choose to get some of their protein requirements from red meat. Many of us have been programmed by family eating habits, advertising, and clever packaging to enjoy meat—for we certainly are not instinctually meat eaters, as are wolves, dogs, lions, and other carnivorous species. We certainly do not drool over dead animals on the side of the road, nor do we naturally get pleasure from the sound of an animal getting ripped apart as do carnivores. We also do not gravitate towards raw flesh. Animals in the wild do get this pleasure naturally, because they are genetically and physically designed for it. In fact, our bodies are designed much more like plant eaters than carnivores. We are almost identical to plant eaters. Cavemen were not the most nutritionally educated people on the planet in my opinion, but I have heard more than once from people that they eat meat because they believe that since the cavemen ate meat, it must be good for us. Cavemen probably just copied what their animal friends did, using survival instincts—not because they were designed to eat meat. It is this survival instinct inside us, as well as the fact that we have been programmed to accept the sight of a well-packaged piece of meat which is then cooked and flavored, that has gravitated humans towards being meat eaters.

If people are to eat meat, they simply need to realize that the body will use many more times the amount of energy to digest the meat, because of the length of the digestive system, the small amount of digestive enzymes and hydrochloric acid as compared to animals, and the acidic nature of meat, which has been proven to cause inflammation. In fact, it has been proven that arthritic conditions in prehistoric times started when man started to eat meat.

Even though I do not recommend eating meat, if you are going to eat meat, you simply have to have an awareness so you can take actions to reduce the harmful effects that meat eating has over the long term (certainly not in the short term, which is why it is transparent and not obvious). Here are some suggestions I give to people who are meat-eating athletes that you could use as a guide.

1. I wouldn't eat meat within forty-eight hours of competition. It takes a few days for meat to pass through the twenty feet of digestive tract.
2. It would help your enzyme factory to take enzyme supplements (proteases, e.g., bromelain and papain; amylase; and lipase).
3. Eat more raw food than you are eating meat. Eat a huge salad which contains active enzymes, and add avocado and olive oil, which contain lipase and will help break down the fats in the meat.
4. Take probiotics (good bacteria) to help the intestinal flora fight off any bacteria in the flesh of the meat.

5. Eat organic, free-range meats. Organic meats mean that the animal is fed organic food and is allowed to roam free and eat mineral-rich grasses. The animal is not fed any hormones, antibiotics, or pesticides and is therefore happier. The happier the animal, the cleaner and more life energy will be in the meat.

I know that most people eat meat out of habit and that probably more than 25 percent would not eat it if they had all the facts. I understand the saying, "What you don't know won't hurt you." However, when it comes to food, that is simply not true. I have best friends that still tell me when I eat a salad that it is going to kill me. They say that we were meant to eat meat because cavemen ate meat; yet they are seventy pounds overweight. This is just an example of the way the majority of the population approaches their food choices.

There are beliefs and assumptions in our minds that were planted there along the way. Throw in the human ego and our natural need to defend our beliefs, and it is very difficult to accept additional education. It usually takes some sort of enlightenment which comes about through some sort of major publicized event—such as the recent news (see http://articles.mercola.com) that 140 million pounds of meat was just recalled because of the way animals were fed and treated in a slaughterhouse in California. I predict this is just the beginning of massive amounts of information which will be discovered about the future of food and how the food supply has been compromised by agriculture.

I believe the most critical thing that anyone can do for their diet is to keep an open mind. Realize that something you know may not be correct, because the facts just haven't managed to cross your space, or the facts just are not out there yet and may hit the news tomorrow. We only have as much information as the information which we seek out or which seeks us out. I have resolved to not be set in my ways. If evidence is reported tomorrow that eating meat will help extend our lives to over 125 years old and the source and evidence seems credible to me, I then have something to act on or to not act on. Without the information, all I have is the forces of advertising or the knowledge handed down to me by someone else who may not have had all the facts. The best thing to do is to align yourself with what feels good and what feels right for you. You know whether something is giving you more or less energy, whether it is helping you lose or gain weight, and whether it is making you feel guilt and shame or joy and happiness.

Strength training

Strength training is a critical aspect to our health if we want to stay injury-free, enjoy sports, look good, feel good, and help prevent premature aging. I personally went to a personal trainer course so I could learn how to work out properly. I wanted to get some hands-on training. I learned that there are many ways to build strength. For instance, if you want to build muscular endurance of the chest muscles, you can use several ways to do this. The traditional way is to use a machine by doing a bench press. You can also use your own body's weight and do a push-up. You can use dumbbells, lie on a bench and do flys, or use tension bands. If we do not use our muscles, we lose our muscles. Strength training also has an effect on our metabolism and may help us lose weight. You do not have to work out every day to achieve benefits. Strength training two to three times a week is sufficient for health and to keep the muscles from getting injured during aerobic exercise. When you're incorporating strength training into your aerobic training, you can work out before or after your aerobic training, depending on the intensity of each. Endurance athletes are sometimes too tired after a hard endurance session to work out afterwards, so they can work out before, but warming up is important and slightly stretching is also important before the aerobic work starts.

Get into herbs

Herbs, in particular, have caught my attention because over the years, I have learned that some of these herbs have super qualities and could in fact alter my entire outlook on life by increasing my energy levels to quantum levels. In addition to helping myself, I find myself having a huge impact on other people who are open to hearing about some of these herbs. I attended a San Diego Chargers game not too long ago, and as most people are aware, these games are filled with carnivorous loving fans that tailgate for hours, drinking alcohol and eating pounds of meats and breads. I came across an individual who was a photographer. He was filled with a hunger for life but was low on energy. He had just eaten large quantities of meat, and he in fact was obese and looked older than he actually was. I was eating a bag of goji berries, and I overheard him say he only ate meat for the protein and he in fact did not really care for it. He even felt deep down it was probably bad for him. I told him that the goji berry is one of the most nutritionally rich fruits/herbs on the planet, that it is a complete protein with all the essential amino acids, that it is rich in fiber and trace minerals, that it is a good source of vitamin C and iron, and that it is a great snack food. He had not known that the goji berry even existed and was thrilled to hear that his local health food store carried it. At that moment, he told me he would probably never eat meat again and wanted to learn about other high-protein plant-based foods. This story and many others have been a motivation for me in writing articles and books about superfoods, herbs, and wellness.

There is no mistaking that our modern food supply does not contain the rich nutrients that it once did and that we are bombarded with pharmaceutical remedies for most of our illnesses. I have found many herbs that I believe may have superior medicinal qualities that can lead you to extreme health and towards an abundant, successful life, by increasing your energy and helping your own body prevent you from getting sick. Health has to be a primary objective for yourself. I often tell people who are as confused and unfocused as I was that you have many paths and roads before you which you can choose to take. Yet if the one you choose does not lead you to extreme health, you may have chosen the wrong path. Herbs like the goji berry have been around for thousands of years and have been used in medicine by ancient civilizations to help their kings and queens rid themselves of disease. The goji berry is of particular importance to me because it is one of the first herbs that I saw with Kirlian photography. The goji berry is an herb that has been used in Chinese history for more than five thousand years and is considered one of the top (if not the #1) herb out of eight thousand plus herbs in Chinese herbal medicine. That's a pretty powerful realization!

I have been fascinated with herbs since 1982, when I joined the U.S Marines. I knew that if I was going to complete the rigorous mental and physical training during the heat of the summer in Parris Island, I would have to educate myself about nutrition. I read books on vitamins, minerals, and herbs, and learned about ginseng being great for endurance (see below). Then I visited local health food stores and read all the labels. My diet back then was whatever my family could afford to eat or whatever I could steal. It was not an organic, whole food–based diet. No one back then had that kind of diet as far as I knew. I did not know about the goji berry back when I joined the marines, but I did learn about others which helped me prepare myself for the training I did back then, such as the ginseng. These herbs are not the source of my carbohydrates but are some of the keys to my strong immune system, which takes a huge beating during vigorous exercise.

The second herb is a very well-known herb and it is called ginseng. Ginseng has been a part of Chinese herbal medicine for over five thousand years. Ginseng strengthens the heart and nervous system. It builds resistance to disease by strengthening our immune system and has anticarcinogenic properties. A good-quality ginseng can also provide strength and endurance, which are of particular interest to athletes, including myself.

An interesting story about my top two herbs is of a man from China by the name of Li Chung Yun who lived to be 252 years old. Goji berries and ginseng were part of his daily consumption. He was born in 1678 and died in 1930. When he gave a speech at the University of Beijing, he was around 200 years old.

The third herb is an herb out of Ayurvedic medicine from India called Tulsi. This herb is also called holy basil. I don't know about you, but any herb that is considered a top herb in India is an herb I want to learn more about. There are many people in India that live extremely long lives as a result of taking many herbs, practicing deep breathing, and using meditation techniques. These modalities help relieve stress, oxygenate the body, and keep the mind and soul alive. Holy basil is an adaptogen. I like this in an herb because it helps relieve stress in many parts of the body, depending on where it is needed. It seems to have the intelligence to give me physical strength when I need it, make me think more clearly when I need it, and help me if I'm feeling tired from exercise. There are other adaptogens I take, but this one I like in particular because of its historical context.

Another great herb is one I take a lot of in the winter instead of getting the normal flu shot (as I used to get every year). It is called the Reishi mushroom. I like this in supplemental form because I can add it to smoothies before an event; it supports the immune and respiratory systems. I was one who would get bronchitis every year. When I started eating these herbs, I was able to get through any onset of bronchitis without antibiotics—and that is important to me because antibiotics have been shown to reduce the probiotics (good bacteria) in our intestinal tract.

Another fantastic herb/spice is cinnamon. Cinnamon is known to kill 80 percent of all bacteria, and it has very powerful alkaline properties. Cinnamon is also high in chromium, which may control blood sugar. An increased alkalinity, in my opinion, is one of the keys to the best health ever and the ability to fight off cancers.

There is an herb that comes out of the Amazon called cat's claw that I have learned about recently, and it has a tremendous amount of mood-enhancing properties—though what I like most is its antiviral properties. Anyone who suffers from getting cold sores or viral infections should look for herbs and minerals which are antiviral.

I have to mention black walnut hull as one of my favorites. I first heard of black walnut hull while I was taking Isagenix's cleansing product (see http://www.antiaging.isagenix.com). I researched all the ingredients in Isagenix, and black walnut hull was one that I believe is a key ingredient because of its ability to cleanse out the parasites and toxins in our digestive system. The importance of cleansing is a huge factor in a health and wellness program. You have to unplug all the bad stuff out of you as a first very important step.

Ginger is also one of my favorites. As an athlete, I can experience a tremendous amount of inflammation all over as a result of training. I add gingerroot to my smoothies, and I also take certain supplements which include ginger. I don't believe in having to take over-the-counter anti-inflammatories. There are so many natural anti-inflammatories that inflammation is no longer an issue with keeping myself fit and fighting off illness.

The power of my next herb has been known for centuries. Garlic is awesome. It tastes great in foods, serves as a powerful natural antibiotic, and helps your arteries, your heart, and your lungs. Although garlic has some odors, it can still be consumed once or twice a week at night. The garlic will be out of your system by morning. If it isn't, it could be a sign that it is doing its job to remove toxins which are trying to get the heck out of the way. Another alternative is aged garlic. I love taking aged garlic three or four times a week. It is available in supplemental form. The raw form is more potent, but the aged variety can be added if you would like to consume more of it on a consistent basis.

My last honorable mentions are parsley, oregano, and vanilla. All three of these have been used in cooking and for flavoring for centuries. They are all extremely powerful herbs which support the immune system.

I have concentrated on the few select herbs in my diet which to me are highly available, somewhat well known, and simple to consume. There are thousands of herbs, but there is a lot of redundancy in their benefits. Quite simply, if it is from nature, was put on this planet, and has survived for thousands of years…then it probably has a lot of power in its ability to help us as humans. Most of the benefits of herbs are well known, and some are not. I strongly believe a diet which includes herbs such as the ones mentioned in this book can serve you in your journey towards a long, healthy life!

Get sun every day

Besides getting vitamin D from the sun, which has been proven to help reduce the possibilities of getting many cancers, getting more sun just makes sense. Flowers and plants thrive in the sunlight. Absorbing the sun's rays transfers to us the same life force energy that plants thrive on.

Endurance training

Endurance training can be addictive. I am sure there are physiological reasons for this, such as the release of endorphins, but for me it is the addiction to always feeling and looking good. When we train for endurance, we help our detoxification system, our cardiovascular system, and our circulatory system. Oxygen levels increase in our bloodstream, and our hearts stay strong and healthy. There are many ways to get endurance training, including running, swimming, cycling, soccer, basketball, boxing, wrestling, and tennis. Four to six days a week of endurance training is great for you if you can maintain it.

Understand the difference between fitness and health

We as humans come in all shapes and sizes (short, tall, round, slim, muscular, fat). Even the smallest of people could be extremely strong, and someone overweight is often seen passing someone much thinner in a marathon. Being fit with a low body fat percentage or being able to bench 350 pounds does not necessarily make someone healthy. Fitness, by definition, is the state of being physically active on a regular basis to maintain good physical condition. Healthy, on the other hand, can have several meanings:

- Being free of illness and disease
- Being able to do things well with high spirits and vigor and joy
- Being prosperous and productive in your ways and attitudes

The ideal situation is to achieve both. Having strong muscles or a high capacity of VO2 levels (maximum oxygen consumption) does not mean your digestive system is healthy or your skin is elastic or your immune system is strong. I understand that society in general has not taught us as a mass population to know the difference between the two. At forty-three years old, I still have to consciously and aggressively seek out the information I need on proper ways to exercise, the proper foods to eat, natural sources of healing, and new discoveries in alternative medicine. These nuggets of wisdom will not be on the front page of *The New*

York Times, and they are not taught to every individual, who indeed has a birthright to know. This book is an attempt to deliver some of that information to you.

Reduce electromagnetic pollution

All electric, electronic, and battery-powered devices produce electromagnetic fields, called EMFs. EMFs are disruptive to our body's own natural energy field. When the electromagnetic energies, coupled with all the frequencies from TVs, microwave ovens, satellites, computers, cell phones, power lines, etc., hit the human energy field, they disrupt it, damage it, and interfere with its normal functioning. These disruptive energies eventually take a toll on the physical body: we get headaches, feel tired, and often develop immune system disorders. Explore EMF reduction and grounding devices that are available for your computer and cell phones

Listen to music

There have been numerous studies done on the effects that music has on water crystals and its use for human healing.

Use doctors wisely

If surgery is needed for a major accident, then a doctor is essential; however, for preventative health, I find it better to use naturopathic practitioners that are schooled in nutrition and holistic health.

Avoid foods and substances that may contribute to obesity, heart disease, high cancer rates, and diabetes.

Avoid foods such as fast food; caffeinated beverages; butters; lards; trans fats; partially hydrogenated and fully hydrogenated oils; processed foods and flours; high-fructose corn syrup; aspartame; artificial dyes, colors, and sweeteners; and artificial flavors.

Be careful not to fall into the gene trap

I understand that some people live to ninety that smoke heavily, and others drink wine every day and live to over one hundred. I also understand that some people have a family history of heart disease or cancer. Some people indeed have a true genetic defect that makes them more susceptible to certain ailments. I believe that these defects are the loaded guns, but it is our lifestyle and food choices that ultimately pull the trigger in most cases. For the one guy out of 1 million that has a superior detoxification system and can filter out nicotine and alcohol, there are 999,999 that cannot. As long as you control your own life, there is no excuse. Do not use your family's past or the story you read about the Costa Rican man who smoked till he was one hundred as an excuse to procrastinate taking care of yourself in the ways that you are learning about in this book.

Avoid microwaving

Don't touch that dial!! And I don't mean the dial on your TV, but the dial on your microwave. I have not used a microwave oven in quite some time. When I did use one, I had always had this awkward gut feeling like something was strange about a bright light and a weird wind-like sound that would heat up the food I placed in the microwave. I never liked what I did not understand. I still do not know the technical details behind how a microwave oven works or how it heats food, but what I do know is that to me it feels unnatural.

I have read many claims about the unhealthy nature behind microwave ovens—women that have been killed when their blood was microwaved at a hospital or that baby's milk should not be heated in a microwave; if it's unhealthy for babies, why wouldn't it be unhealthy for adults? Why would certain countries outside the United States ban the use of microwave ovens? I truly believe that heating food with a microwave changes the chemical structure of the food into a structure that the body has to figure out when the food is swallowed. When the body is unable to figure out what to do with the food, it may look at it like a toxin and push it off into a fat cell or rush it through your digestive system as fast as it can to get it out of there since it is unable to absorb the nutrients which it no longer understands.

In 1976, Russia banned the use of microwaves after finding out that there were negative health results in their research. Most of the negativity resulted from the findings surrounding the greater possibility of cancer. Higher percentages of cancerous cells were found in the bloodstream after people ate microwaved foods.

I read about an experiment you can do at home related to raising awareness of the strange effects that microwaving could have on our health. Plant some sprouting seeds in two separate pots, and water one with spring water and the other with microwaved tap water. The plant being fed with microwaved water will not grow. That is an amazing insight as to what microwaving could be doing to our own bodies.

The heating process itself does have damaging consequences to our food. Approximately half the protein is destroyed in the heating process, enzymes are just about completely destroyed, and other valuable nutrients are lost in the process. Add microwaving as your heating source and you now have distorted molecules of what is not destroyed for your digestive system to figure out. I always felt like I was being exposed to radiation whenever I was close to a microwave oven. I would see these microwave testers at the store and say to myself, *Why would we need this if microwaving is not dangerous?* Use your own intuition and be resourceful as to what the harmful effects of microwaving may be. The way I see it is that there are probably much better ways to cook your food if cooking is what makes you happy.

Reduce alcohol intake

Alcohol can be detrimental to your health if not consumed in moderation. There is so much more negative that comes from it than positive in the world, and it certainly undermines the detoxification role that our liver takes on minute by minute. Occasional drinking is fine, because it reduces stress from other areas of your life, and the fun that can come from socializing and making friends is extremely important. Because it is so addictive, however, it can take control of your better judgment and often does. I would say the friends you choose and the lifestyle you choose are very important if this is a problem.

Avoid antibiotics

I understand the urge to take antibiotics at the first sign of a cough or runny nose. Medicines and pills can become very addictive and can become crutches and a substitute for being responsible for our health. I would reach for cold medicines and antibiotics every time I got a slight cough because it was uncomfortable to be sick. Once I started staying more hydrated and drinking strong herbal teas, my immune system got stronger and sickness became less frequent. If I do start to feel less than optimal, it is because I have become dehydrated and did not eat as optimally as I know I could have in the previous days. The effects that processed foods have on your body are much more noticeable once you eliminate them from your diet and then you cheat and add them back.

Avoid carbonated beverages

Carbonated beverages are very acidic and can leach minerals from your system. When I used to drink a lot of carbonated beverages, I seemed to be always popping antacids—not to mention that most soft drinks contain artificial colors, flavors, and sweeteners.

Use natural toothpaste, shampoo, shaving cream, mouthwash, body lotions, makeups, soaps, cleaners, and detergents.

Everything that touches your skin can make its way into your pores and bloodstream. The more organic and natural the substances you use for everyday body care and cleaning of your clothes and household, the fewer chemicals will make their way into your pores. Household cleaners evaporate and get trapped in well-insulated houses.

Use natural sweeteners and avoid artificial sweeteners

Blue agave nectar, stevia, honey, and yacon root syrup are natural sweeteners; aspartame and sucralose are artificial sweeteners.

Foods for the immune system

Foods for the immune system include Reishi mushrooms, cordyceps, shiitake mushrooms, garlic, onions, apples, turmeric, oregano, green tea, leafy greens, and vitamin C–rich foods.

Athlete special

As an Ironman athlete, I am always thinking of what I can do to have the best health ever. I want to have the most energy, recover quickly, prevent destructive oxidative damage, keep stress levels low, keep my joints healthy, keep overall inflammation low, keep my digestive system healthy so I can absorb nutrients better during training, and keep hydrated. I follow the advice and eating habits as closely as possible that I have described in this book. I want to list the key foods, however, and the key nutrients that I take.

Main "staple" foods

- Quinoa
- Fruits: bananas, grapes, apples, pears, berries, cherries, bananas, oranges

- Salads (kale, iceberg lettuce, spinach leaves, romaine, olives, nuts, seeds, tomatoes, cucumbers, peppers, sea salt, avocados, celery)
- Olive oil, flaxseed oil, hemp oil, grape seed oil
- Smoothies:

    The primary content varies depending on the day but consists of some of the following:

    Cacao, maca powder, seeds (pumpkin, sunflower, sesame, flax), nuts (walnuts, almonds), hemp protein, hemp seeds, cordyceps, bananas, frozen berries, calcium, vitamin D and magnesium powder, powdered fruit and berries or raw and fresh if available, green superfood powder, protein superfood powder, grass powder, bee pollen
    The base of the smoothie is one or more of the following:

    Water, orange juice, rice milk, oat milk, almond milk, hemp milk

Supplemental foods

These are foods that come in capsule or droplet form which I will take during intense training, when I am cleansing, when I am traveling, when I am low on whole raw foods around the house, when I need a boost to my immune system, or when I just feel like taking them with a smoothie:

marine phytoplankton, zeolites immune detox, collodial gold, CoQ_{10}, juice plus™, aloe vera, organic MSM (Methylsulfonylmethane), beauty enzymes from www.Sunfood.

com, fiber with probiotics, and tissue rejuvenator from hammer nutrition, revitaphi, wheatgrass, organic bars

Pre-workout nutrition

Smoothie: blended oats, banana , hemp, agave, rice, oat or hemp milk, spiz liquid nutrition, water

Other: I prefer liquid nutrition; however, I will sometimes go with whole grain sprouted toast with organic jelly, organic pancakes

Bike nutrition

Spiz liquid nutrition, blended dates, coconut water and oil, blended hemp seed, high pH water

Run nutrition

Hammer gels, spiz liquid nutrition, raw food available on run course (banana, orange)

Post-workout nutrition

Within ten minutes of end of workout: water
Then: raw food carbohydrates (banana, orange, apple)
Then: within thirty minutes of end of workout: carb protein blended smoothie or powder recovery drink (4 to 1 carb to protein ratio)
Within ninety minutes of end of workout or race: complex carbs and protein meal

Antioxidant nutrition for athletes to combat oxidative stress:

Grape seed extract; green tea; L-glutathione; vitamins A, C, and E; alpha lipoic acid; N-acetyl cysteine; polyphenol-rich foods (cacao, grapes, blueberries, broccoli, apples, onions); Juice Plus™; CoQ_{10}; extra virgin olive oil; goji berries

Anti-inflammatory nutrition for swelling:

For me, I consider to be among the best natural anti-inflammatories: turmeric, omega 3's, organic MSM, ginger, boswelllia, enzymes (papain and bromelain), olive oil, krill oil, aloe vera, hemp seed, and vitamin C–rich foods.

Drink the super juices

These include noni juice, acai juice, mangosteen juice, pomegranate juice, and aloe vera juice.

Eat fruits, melons, and berries

These include Inca berries, goji berries, raspberries, strawberries, blueberries, watermelon, apples, grapes, plums, bananas, and pineapple.

Eat cucumbers, peppers, and tomatoes

I call these the "seed fruits," and they are great for healthy snacking.

Eat super omega-3-rich foods

These include olives, avocados, flaxseeds, hemp seeds, marine phytoplankton, salmon, walnuts, chia seeds, almonds, and krill oil.

Eat super herbs and spices

These include holy basil, ginseng, cat's claw, pau d'arco, cinnamon, parsley, oregano, turmeric, cayenne, ginger, ginko biloba, ho shu wu, and ashwaganda. (All of these could just be added in small amounts to a smoothie, which is why smoothies are so great and powerful. Most people add spices to cooked foods, which diminishes their nutritional value significantly.)

Consume antiaging foods

These include leafy greens, berries, green tea, resveratrol (found in grapes, red wine, mulberries, and peanuts), spices and herbs, coconut oil, water, avocados, cacao, garlic, onions, olive oil, nuts, seeds, and tomatoes.

Consume longevity foods

These include ginseng, goji berries, coconut oil, green tea, turmeric, flaxseeds, olives, leafy greens, berries, oats, cacao, sea vegetables, garlic, apples, onions, tomatoes, and nuts.

Take stress-relieving foods/herbs when needed

There are foods and herbs which are well know as natural stress relievers, such as rhodiola, colloidal gold, maca, ashwaganda, cordyceps, and ginseng.

Discuss getting routine tests with your naturopathic practitioner

These include eye and ear exams, testing your vitamin and mineral levels, testing your amino acid levels, checking your thyroid levels, checking your PSA, checking your cholesterol, checking your neurotransmitters, and doing a stool test. Also, do a blood profile (see below), urine profile, bone density test, and possibly an ultrafast CT scan if your doctor suggest it (if you are worried about artery clogs; may need an MD to order this exam).

Consider a Comprehensive Blood Profile

The Biophysical 250 (http://www.biophysicalcorp.com) surveys the biomarkers in your blood that could indicate many conditions and diseases, including:

> Cardiovascular disease (such as risk for heart attack and stroke)
> Cancer (including breast, colon, liver, ovarian, prostate, and pancreatic)
> Metabolic disorders (such as diabetes and metabolic syndrome)
> Autoimmune disease (including rheumatoid arthritis and lupus)
> Viral and bacterial diseases (such as mononucleosis and pneumonia)
> Hormonal imbalance (including menopause, testosterone deficiency, thyroid deficiency)
> Nutritional status (such as vitamin deficiencies, protein deficiencies)

Get your genetic profile (e.g., www.23andme.com)

With a 23andMe gene profile, you can discover how your genes influence your health and traits. You can get your data on over ninety traits and diseases. Trace your maternal line using mitochondrial DNA. Trace your paternal line via the Y chromosome. Identify the region or regions where the majority of your ancestors likely originated using global similarity. There are also sports varieties of gene testing that will analyze genes involved in cardiovascular endurance and strength, which can recommend different nutritional remedies based on your athletic potential.

Shower filter

We bathe every day, and the chemicals that come out of our shower get absorbed through the skin. Weigh yourself on a scale that goes to the tenth of a pound. Stand in the shower for ten minutes, dry off, and weigh yourself after, and you will be surprised that you have gained weight from the absorption of the water. Investing in a shower filter can be a wise choice in eliminating some of this toxic absorption.

Cigarettes, cigars, chewing

The products themselves say right on the packaging that the surgeon general advises that the product will cause cancer.

Silvertooth fillings (which contain mercury)

Mercury evaporates from old-style fillings that many of us received as kids. Mercury is a poisonous substance.

Eat more raw and fewer cooked foods

Our bodies produce a white blood cell response when we eat more cooked foods than raw food in a particular meal. Eating more raw food than cooked food (more than 50 percent) does not produce this white blood cell response. I believe this is because the body can use the enzymes effectively in the raw food to handle the digestion of the food.

Black walnut hull

This is a great herb which can be used for getting rid of parasites in the digestive tract.

Other tips which may increase your life span (and mine)

- Have lots of friends
- Participate in dangerous sports wisely
- Drive safely
- Floss
- Stretch daily
- Consider CoQ_{10} supplementation; it reduces in quantity in our cells as we age
- Discuss with your naturopath taking calcium, vitamin D3, and magnesium as supplements (these are some of the most deficient minerals in humans)
- Oxygenate your house with plants such as aloe vera, Chinese evergreens, and spider plants
- Change the type of salt you use from processed to Celtic sea salt or Himalayan salt
- Determine your metabolic type (some people thrive on higher-protein, -fat, or -carb diets because of the makeup of their mitochondria)

- Eat lightly, several times a day, mostly plants
- Volunteer and stay active as you age
- Explore meditation and yoga
- Have the most awesome days (and nights) ever

Me: Hey have I seen you before?
Girl: No, Why?
Me: Cause I was looking a dictionary the other day and saw the word beautiful